Research and Perspectives in Endocrine Interactions

More information about this series at http://www.springer.com/series/5241

Bruce Spiegelman
Editor

Hormones, Metabolism and the Benefits of Exercise

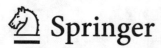 Springer

Editor
Bruce Spiegelman
Dana-Farber Cancer Institute
Harvard Medical School
Boston, MA
USA

Fondation IPSEN
Boulogne-Billancourt
France

Acknowledgement: The editors wish to express their gratitude to Mrs. Mary Lynn Gage for her editorial assistance.

ISSN 1861-2253   ISSN 1863-0685   (electronic)
Research and Perspectives in Endocrine Interactions
ISBN 978-3-030-10268-5   ISBN 978-3-319-72790-5   (eBook)
https://doi.org/10.1007/978-3-319-72790-5

Printed on acid-free paper

This Springer imprint is published by Springer Nature
The registered company is Springer International Publishing AG
The registered company address is: Gewerbestrasse 11, 6330 Cham, Switzerland

Preface

We gathered in Paris to present new work on exercise and the molecular understanding of its actions and benefits. Exercise has been understood for centuries to provide benefits to the human body. Diet and exercise have long been prescribed as the first lines of therapy for metabolic diseases such as obesity and type 2 diabetes. However, it is perhaps not fully appreciated that exercise is also effective at improving the function of the liver, muscles themselves, and (importantly) the brain. Endurance exercise is one of the only ways that adult humans can stimulate de novo neurogenesis. If we can understand the precise ways that these benefits occur, we can hope to both optimize exercise protocols and perhaps find molecular entities that can bring benefits beyond what can be done by exercise alone.

It is critical to note that the goal of most basic scientists in this area is *not* to replace exercise with a pill. Indeed, this seems a very naïve and unlikely goal. However, it is important to recognize that many people cannot exercise effectively because of age or infirmities such as cancer, neuromuscular diseases, neurodegeneration, and postsurgical trauma. Furthermore, there is a limit to how much exercise even fit people can do, as exercise takes time and can itself be associated with joint or muscle inflammation. Perhaps specific molecules regulated in exercise can be dosed well beyond what is naturally produced during exercise. While this idea is still at the hypothetical stage, the NIH has responded to these challenges and opportunities by launching the new program "Molecular Transducers of Physical Activity."

Exercise is not one thing. It can differ in duration, intensity, and type of activity. Running and weight lifting are very different things, and they are likely to involve different signaling systems and bring different benefits. The response to exercise also has a time element: short-term studies might show a degree of tissue damage, whereas longer term studies are more likely to show benefits.

Our own work in this area was stimulated by the observations made by us and others that the transcriptional coactivator PGC1α, which we discovered in brown fat, is induced in muscle with endurance training; it then stimulates mitochondrial biogenesis and many of the pathways seen in endurance-trained muscle. Included here was an observed resistance to muscular dystrophy and muscle atrophy, at least in mice. Our interest in how PGC1α expression in muscle leads to benefits in distant tissues led to the discovery of irisin, a small secreted protein derived from muscle (a "myokine") that is controlled by exercise and PGC1α in mice and humans.

With this as background, this volume contains new work presented at this conference that attempts to expand the dialogue between scientists focused on human exercise studies and those who want to understand these processes at the molecular level. Surely, our ability to develop new therapies in this area will require close collaborations between academics and eventually with the biotech and pharmaceutical worlds.

Dana-Farber Cancer Institute   Bruce Spiegelman
Harvard Medical School
Boston, MA, USA

Contents

List of Contributors

Claude Bouchard Human Genomics Laboratory, Pennington Biomedical Research Center, Baton Rouge, LA, USA

School of Nutrition, Laval University, Quebec City, QC, Canada

Francesco S. Celi Division of Endocrinology Diabetes and Metabolism, Department of Internal Medicine, Virginia Commonwealth University, Richmond, VA, USA

Regula Furrer Biozentrum, University of Basel, Basel, Switzerland

Christoph Handschin Biozentrum, University of Basel, Basel, Switzerland

John A. Hawley Mary MacKillop Institute for Health Research, Australian Catholic University, Melbourne, VIC, Australia

Research Institute for Sport and Exercise Sciences, Liverpool John Moores University, Liverpool, UK

Zihong He Human Genomics Laboratory, Pennington Biomedical Research Center, Baton Rouge, LA, USA

Department of Biology, China Institute of Sport Science, Beijing, China

Mohammad Rashedul Islam Massachussetts General Hospital and Harvard Medical School, Charlestown, MA, USA

Anna Krook Department of Physiology and Pharmacology, Integrative Physiology, Karolinska Institutet, Stockholm, Sweden

Arthur S. Leon Department of Biology, China Institute of Sport Science, Beijing, China

Magnus Lindgren Niss Department of Physiology and Pharmacology, Integrative Physiology, Karolinska Institutet, Stockholm, Sweden

Tuomo Rankinen Human Genomics Laboratory, Pennington Biomedical Research Center, Baton Rouge, LA, USA

Jorge Lira Ruas Department of Physiology and Pharmacology, Molecular and Cellular Exercise Physiology, Karolinska Institutet, Stockholm, Sweden

Rasmus J. O. Sjögren Department of Molecular Medicine and Surgery, Karolinska Institutet, Stockholm, Sweden

James S. Skinner School of Kinesiology, University of Minnesota, Minneapolis, MN, USA

Bruce Spiegelman Dana-Farber Cancer Institute, Harvard Medical School, Boston, MA, USA

André Tchernof Department of Kinesiology, Indiana University, Bloomington, IN, USA

Paula Valente-Silva Department of Physiology and Pharmacology, Molecular and Cellular Exercise Physiology, Karolinska Institutet, Stockholm, Sweden

Benoit Viollet Institut Cochin, INSERM, U1016, Paris, France

CNRS, UMR8104, Paris, France

Université Paris Descartes, Sorbonne Paris cité, Paris, France

Christiane D. Wrann Massachussetts General Hospital and Harvard Medical School, Charlestown, MA, USA

Michael F. Young Massachussetts General Hospital and Harvard Medical School, Charlestown, MA, USA

Human Brown Adipose Tissue Plasticity: Hormonal and Environmental Manipulation

Francesco S. Celi

Abstract Brown adipose tissue (BAT), brown-in-white ("brite") and "beige" adipocytes share the unique ability of converting chemical energy into heat and play a critical role in the adaptive thermogenesis response promoting nonshivering thermogenesis. Uncoupling Protein-1 (UCP1), which allows the uncoupling of substrate oxidation from phosphorylation of ADP, represents the molecular signature of BAT and beige adipocytes. Until recently, the physiologic role of BAT and beige adipocytes depots was thought to be limited to small mammalians and newborns.

The discovery of BAT in adult humans and the demonstration of the presence of inducible BAT activity in white adipose tissue by beige adipocytes have generated enthusiasm as potential targets for treatment of obesity and other disorders due to sustained positive energy balance. These findings are particularly important since in vitro studies have demonstrated that preadipocytes can be directed toward a common brown phenotype by multiple pathways that, in turn, may be exploited for therapeutic interventions. In adult humans, BAT activity is more evident in deep neck fat depots and, to a lesser degree, in subcutaneous adipose tissue, with a transcriptome signature resembling the rodent beige fat. This observation supports the hypothesis that human BAT activity and capacity can be modulated. To this end, we have directed our translational research program toward the characterization of beige fat in humans and on the effects of hormonal and environmental drivers in the adaptive thermogenesis response. Mild cold exposure, within the temperature range commonly employed in climate-controlled buildings, is sufficient to generate a significant increase in non-shivering thermogenesis driven by BAT and beige adipocyte activation. In turn, adaptive thermogenesis generates a specific hormonal signature and promotes glucose disposal. Chronic exposure to mild cold induces expansion of BAT mass and activity, whereas exposure to warm climate abrogates them. Additionally, the metabolic effects of BAT mass expansion are evident only upon stimulation of BAT activity, indicating that both

F. S. Celi (✉)
Division of Endocrinology Diabetes and Metabolism, Department of Internal Medicine, Virginia Commonwealth University, Richmond, VA, USA
e-mail: Francesco.celi@vchuhealth.org

© The Author(s) 2017
B. Spiegelman (ed.), *Hormones, Metabolism and the Benefits of Exercise*,
Research and Perspectives in Endocrine Interactions,
https://doi.org/10.1007/978-3-319-72790-5_1

expansion and activation of BAT are necessary and complementary strategies to pursue. From an experimental standpoint, human preadipocytes represent a viable experimental platform to mechanistically interrogate different pathways that are able to expand and activate browning. Our laboratory has focused on studying FGF-21, and FNDC5/irisin in their capacity to promote the browning process. Compared to a white differentiation medium, the addition of either FGF-21 or FNDC5 results in a reprogramming toward a brown phenotype, as indicated by the display of brown transcriptome signature and, functionally, by the increase in oxygen consumption following catecholamine treatment, indicating an increase in substrate utilization. Collectively, the integration of a detailed assessment of human physiology with mechanistic observations in cell culture systems can provide a unique opportunity to translate observations from experimental models to actionable therapeutic targets.

Introduction

The unique ability of mammalians (and to some degree avians; Vianna et al. 2001) to maintain their core temperature independently of the environmental temperature has allowed their evolutionary success and, compared to poikilothermic species, to the wide distribution of species across climates. This response is defined as "adaptive thermogenesis," which describes the concerted physiologic responses aimed at defending the core temperature from low environmental temperatures, preserving the individual's ideal core temperature for biologic functions (Stocks et al. 2004). The main components of this response are thermal insulation, non-shivering thermogenesis, and shivering thermogenesis (Celi et al. 2015). From an evolutionary perspective, the excess of energy expenditure aimed at maintaining the core temperature represents a tradeoff between survival and maintenance of energy stores, since the availability of energy usually represents the limiting factor to growth and reproduction for organisms. To this end, moving from an insulative response, which is energy neutral, to a non-shivering and eventually shivering thermogenesis will require a progressively greater dissipation of energy stores (Fig. 1). Additionally, the relative size of the organism and the presence of fur dictate the relative importance of the insulative versus thermogenic response, with smaller organisms being biased toward the latter because of their high surface area-to-volume ratio, which, despite the presence of optimal insulation, will still promote thermal dispersion (Phillips and Heath 1995). Hence, modulation of energy expenditure plays a critical role in the maintenance of core temperature in small mammalians (Ravussin and Galgani 2011). Compared to humans, the capacity of adaptive thermogenesis in small rodents is significantly greater, resulting in an at least twofold increase in total energy expenditure, thus enabling survival in a cold environment, albeit at a price of a compensatory increase in food intake (Ravussin et al. 2014). Over the recent

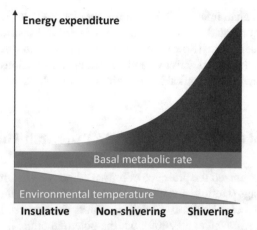

Adaptive thermogenesis response components

Fig. 1 Model of adaptive thermogenesis. As the environmental temperature decreases from thermoneutrality, the adaptive thermogenesis response moves from insulative to non-shivering and eventually shivering thermogenesis. This progression is mirrored by an increase in the energy expenditure required to maintain the core temperature. Green, energy expenditure due to basal metabolic rate; red, expenditure due to adaptive thermogenesis

evolutionary development of the species, humans have gained the ability to modulate their environment using garments and climate-controlled buildings. As a result, exposure to cold is a relatively unusual condition for them and, unless acclimated, individuals tend to respond by shivering thermogenesis, whereby heat is a side product of uncontrolled muscle fasciculation. Of interest, upon prolonged exposure to cold, individuals become resilient and do not display shivering thermogenesis (Davis 1961), indicating that other mechanisms are recruited.

BAT and the Adaptive Thermogenesis Response

BAT has the unique capability of converting energy stores into heat by virtue of the Uncoupling Protein 1 (UCP1), which promotes a proton leak in the inner membrane of the mitochondria, dissociating the oxidative phosphorylation of substrate from the generation of ATP. This process in essence shunts the chemical energy into heat, which is in turn dissipated in the circulation (Nedergaard et al. 2001). The rapid activation and inactivation of the UCP1-driven energy dissipation thus represents a valuable mechanism that is able to increase efficiently the metabolic rate on demand by non-shivering thermogenesis, ultimately promoting the survival of the organism against unfavorable environmental conditions with the least possible consumption of energy stores (Celi 2009).

Aside from the anatomically defined intrascapular BAT, in mice non-shivering thermogenesis is generated in other adipose tissue depots, in particular inguinal, by "beige" or "brown-in-white (brite)" adipocytes (Ishibashi and Seale 2010; Petrovic et al. 2010), whose mass and activity can be modulated by various signal hormones and cytokines, showing a remarkable plasticity (Diaz et al. 2014).

Implications of the Rediscovery of BAT in Adult Humans

Several reports recognized the presence of brown adipocytes in adult humans, either as incidental findings (Huttunen et al. 1981) or as a nuisance in the interpretation of ^{18}F fluorodeoxyglucose Positron Emission Tomography (^{18}F FDG-PET) scans (Hany et al. 2002; Agrawal et al. 2009), but the potential clinical relevance of these findings was missed until the "rediscovery" of BAT. Three manuscripts published in the same issue of the New England Journal of Medicine, from the USA (Cypess et al. 2009), Finland (Virtanen et al. 2009), and the Netherlands (van Marken Lichtenbelt et al. 2009), and followed shortly by a manuscript from Japan (Saito et al. 2009), clearly indicated that BAT was present in a significant number of adults and that its presence and activity (measured by proxy as ^{18}F FDG uptake by PET scanning) correlated with indices of healthy metabolism. Conversely, obesity, diabetes and age inversely correlated with BAT activity (Pfannenberg et al. 2010). Although the initial observations were purely correlative, the potential of a novel therapeutic target for the treatment of the metabolic consequences of obesity led to intense research to expand the capacity and activity of human BAT. Importantly, the location of adult BAT is different from the intrascapular depots observed in newborns (Drubach et al. 2011), and the transcriptome signature resembles more closely the one observed in rodent inguinal fat (Shinoda et al. 2015). This observation is relevant from the therapeutic perspective because of the exquisite plasticity of inguinal adipocytes, providing the rationale to exploit pathways to increase non-shivering thermogenesis as a means of promoting energy disposal with consequent amelioration of obesity and its metabolic consequences.

Integrative Physiology Studies of Human Adaptive Thermogenesis

To better characterize the relevance of the adaptive thermogenesis response, several integrative physiology studies were carried out in humans, mostly by exposing volunteers to cold. While a short but intense cold exposure (such as immersion of a limb in ice-cold water) is able to generate maximal ^{18}F FDG-PET uptake and a significant increase in energy expenditure (Yoneshiro et al. 2011), this method does not correspond to day-to-day experience and cannot be sustained over time.

Table 1 Hormonal axes and organ-system response to mild cold exposure

Hormonal axes and organ systems	Response to cold
Sympathetic nervous system	↑↑
Adrenals (medulla, epinephrine)	↑
Adrenal (cortical, cortisol)	↑
Thyroid axis	↑↔
Fasting glucose	↔
Postprandial glucose	↓
Subcutaneous adipose tissue glucose	↔↓
Fasting insulin	↑
Postprandial insulin	↔
Free fatty acids	↑↑
Subcutaneous adipose tissue lipolysis	↔↑
FGF-21	↑↑

Additionally, intense cold exposure results in muscle fasciculation, with consequential recruitment of shivering thermogenesis. Conversely, mild cold exposure within the thermal envelope of climate-controlled buildings can stimulate a sustained physiologic adaptive thermogenesis response. In a crossover study, the adaptive thermogenesis response to minimal changes in environmental temperature was assessed in healthy volunteers who underwent two 12-h energy expenditure (EE) recordings in a whole room calorimeter (Metabolic Chamber) at 19 and 24 °C (Celi et al. 2010). The system employed in these studies recorded real-time measurements of EE and substrate utilization (respiratory quotient) while sealed ports allowed blood sampling during the study. Moreover, study volunteers were fitted with linear accelerometers and subcutaneous abdominal tissue extracellular fluid microdialysis sampling, and received a standard meal after 6 h of recording, enabling a comprehensive assessment of the physiologic response to short-term mild cold exposure. This complex experimental design allowed to obtain a comprehensive assessment of the physiology of adaptive thermogenesis.

The data obtained from these studies indicated that a minimal modulation of the environmental temperature was sufficient to increase EE by approximately 6%, which corresponds, if projected over 24 h, to 100 kcal in an individual of 70–80 kg. The magnitude of this change may appear insignificant—only one fifth of the negative energy balance recommended to achieve sustained weight loss—but it is important to note that, over a 1-year period (all things being equal), these differences would be equivalent to a 20-day fast and to a daily 30-min walk at a moderate pace. Importantly, these observations also demonstrated that the adaptive thermogenesis response during mild cold exposure resulted in a significant and potentially relevant metabolic effect. A summary of the findings is reported in Table 1 (Celi et al. 2010). Exposure to mild cold is sufficient to drive an adrenergic response, which promotes lipolysis and increased postprandial glucose disposal. The significant lipolysis observed during non-shivering thermogenesis is in keeping with a functional imaging study that demonstrated that fatty acids represent the preferred substrate in BAT depots. On the other hand, the intervention was also sufficient to generate an increase in cortisol and a state of relative insulin resistance during fasting, which indicate an activation of the stress response.

A subsequent study correlated the individual's BAT activity, as measured by ^{18}F FDG uptake in the thoracic region, where BAT is commonly observed with the adaptive thermogenesis response, to mild cold exposure (Chen et al. 2013). In this case, scans were acquired after a 12-h metabolic chamber recording either at 19 or 24 °C and the EE recordings were performed overnight to allow ^{18}F FDG-PET the following morning. By comparing the tracer uptake of the two images, the overall uptake in the region of interest could be calculated and used as a linear variable to be included in multivariate statistical analyses. This strategy provided the opportunity to explore non-shivering thermogenesis as a diffuse function rather than localized in nests of brown adipocytes, overcoming the signal-to-noise ratio limitation of functional imaging. In turn, this variable was used to correlate BAT activity with metabolic and anthropometric parameters. This analysis demonstrated that BAT activity strongly correlated with the increase in EE during mild cold exposure. Remarkably, the association was present in individuals both with and without visible BAT depots on conventional ^{18}F FDG PET imaging, indicating that diffuse (i.e., beige adipocytes-driven) uncoupling activity is an important mediator of non-shivering thermogenesis in adult humans (Chen et al. 2013).

Intervention Studies Aimed to Modulate the Human Adaptive Thermogenesis Response

These correlative studies did not address the question whether human BAT (and beige adipocytes) had the plasticity displayed by murine inguinal fat-depots, or if the capacity of BAT was sufficient to modulate a clinically significant endpoint. A short-term, moderate (10 days acclimatization with exposure at 17 °C daily for 2 h) cold exposure was sufficient to increase BAT as measured by ^{18}F FDG-PET (van der Lans et al. 2013), whereas a similar protocol carried out for a longer period of time (6 weeks acclimatization with exposure at 17 °C daily for 2 h) resulted in significant fat mass reduction (Yoneshiro et al. 2013). In a longer study, the plasticity of the adaptive thermogenesis response was assessed by modulating the environmental temperature overnight (Lee et al. 2014b). Study volunteers were exposed over a period of four consecutive months to 24 °C (run-in period), 19 °C (cold acclimatization), 24 °C (wash-out period), and 30 °C (heat acclimatization). At the end of each month the adaptive thermogenesis response was studied using two consecutive metabolic chamber recordings at 19 and 24 °C; ^{18}F FDG-PET for visualization and measurement of BAT activity was performed after the completion of the 19 °C metabolic chamber stay. After a month-long exposure to mild cold, BAT volume and activity nearly doubled when compared to the end of the run-in period.

Conversely, BAT activity was negligible following a 1-month exposure to warm temperature (30 °C). Remarkably, the increase in BAT activity following the cold acclimatization was accompanied by a significant increase in postprandial glucose disposal, but only during mild cold exposure (Lee et al. 2014b). Thus, the data indicate that human BAT is exquisitely plastic but also that activation (i.e., cold exposure or other pharmacologic means) is necessary to generate a significant metabolic signature.

Collectively, these integrative physiology observations indicate that human BAT and beige depots represent an ideal pharmacologic target for the treatment of the consequences of a sustained positive energy balance because of their plasticity and ability to modulate carbohydrate metabolism.

Manipulation of the Human Adaptive Thermogenesis Response by Hormones and Myokines

Similarly to white adipocytes, BAT and beige adipocytes are not only targets of hormones and cytokines but also have an endocrine function, and their secretome can act in a paracrine and endocrine fashion (Ni et al. 2015). Primary cultures of preadipocytes derived from the stromal vascular fraction of adipose tissues have been proven to be a robust experimental model to assess the effects of hormones and cytokines on their differentiation and function (Diaz et al. 2014). Preadipocytes can be directed toward a white or beige phenotype by hormonal manipulation of the culture media, indirectly demonstrating the plasticity of adipose tissue depots. Moreover, individual hormones, cytokines or drugs can be tested for their ability to promote "beige-ing" in white-differentiating preadipocytes. Our laboratory has worked toward defining the role of two regulators of beige adipocytes, FGF-21 and FNDC5/irisin. FGF-21 is a pleiotropic hormone that is mainly secreted by the liver and promotes insulin sensitization and browning of adipose tissue depots. Interestingly, FGF-21 is also secreted by beige adipocytes, creating an autocrine/ paracrine loop (Ni et al. 2015). In humans, FGF-21 follows a circadian rhythm that is disrupted by cold exposure (Lee et al. 2013). Compared to exposure to 24 °C, exposure to mild cold resulted in an increase in the FGF-21. Importantly, the increase in FGF-21 (compared to thermoneutrality) correlated with the non-shivering thermogenesis response; this finding was also confirmed by measuring the changes in FGF-21 in relation to the lipolysis measured in the subcutaneous adipose tissue mocrodialysate (Lee et al. 2013). Collectively these observations support the role of FGF-21 in promoting and sustaining the adipocyte role in the non-shivering thermogenesis response. When FGF-21 was added to the white differentiating culture medium, human preadipocytes were directed toward a brown phenotype and were able to increase their oxygen consumption and heat production in response to norepinephrine treatment (Lee et al. 2013). These findings recapitulate the clinical observations that FGF-21 plays a pivotal role in beige adipocyte differentiation and function. Unfortunately, therapeutic use of FGF-21 has been limited because of concerns for off-target effects (Kharitonenkov and Adams 2014) possibly due to the systemic administration of the hormone in pharmacologic doses, unlike the local, paracrine action within the adipose tissue depots.

The discovery that BAT derives from a myf-5-positive precursor common to myocytes (Seale et al. 2008) has brought to the forefront the cross-talk between skeletal muscle and brown-beige adipocytes. Similar to adipose tissue depots, skeletal muscle has the ability to secrete myokines with hormonal activity on distant tissues. In particular, Irisin, a fibronectin-like peptide released by skeletal muscle upon contraction, has the ability to promote beige-ing in mouse inguinal adipose tissue depots and to positively affect energy and carbohydrate metabolism (Bostrom et al. 2012). The action of Irisin might appear counterintuitive since it is released by an energy-dissipating organ (skeletal muscle during contraction) and its action promotes the expansion of another energy-dissipating organ tissue (beige adipocytes). On the other hand, this apparent paradox can be reconciled once it is observed from the evolutionary perspective of energy conservation: severe cold exposure, which is able to generate shivering (highly energy inefficient) thermogenesis, promotes the expansion of the capacity of the more energy-efficient BAT and beige adipocyte-driven non-shivering thermogenesis. An integrated physiology experiment was thus designed to evaluate this hypothesis by characterizing the entire spectrum of the adaptive thermogenesis response in healthy volunteers exposed to progressively lower temperatures delivered by cooling blankets (Lee et al. 2014c). This strategy allowed to capture in the same individual the vasoconstrictive response as well non-shivering and shivering thermogenesis, while the EE was annotated by indirect calorimetry (ventilated hood). Study volunteers also underwent basal and post-exercise blood sampling following a maximal exercise tolerance test (VO_2 Max) lasting approximately 15 min and a 60-min resistance exercise at 40% VO_2 Max. The findings of this study demonstrated a large inter-individual variability in both onset of shivering and Irisin secretion either following exercise or during controlled cooling. Furthermore, during cold exposure the release of Irisin was proportional to the shivering intensity (measured by surface electromyography). Interestingly, short-term shivering was sufficient to stimulate the release of a similar amount of Irisin when compared to maximal or resistance exercise (Lee et al. 2014c). When tested on human preadipocytes undergoing white differentiation, Irisin promoted a beige phenotype not dissimilar to the one observed following FGF-21 treatment (Lee et al. 2014a). Collectively these data confirm the role of Irisin as a myokine that is able to expand beige adipocyte mass, increasing the non-shivering thermogenesis capacity and thus promoting a shift from an inefficient (shivering) to a more efficient and sustainable form of thermogenesis (Fig. 2).

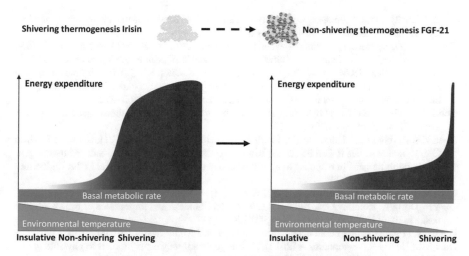

Fig. 2 Model of interplay between shivering and non-shivering thermogenesis. Exposure to cold promotes shivering in non-acclimated individuals, with release of Irisin. This response is costly from an energy-conservation perspective and not sustainable. Irisin promotes the expansion and differentiation of beige adipocytes, which increase resilience to cold enhancing non-shivering thermogenesis and delay the onset of shivering. The greater beige adipocyte mass self-sustains by the autocrine-paracrine effects of FGF-21

Conclusions

In conclusion, human integrated physiology observations coupled with translational studies offer the possibility to explore the potential therapeutic exploitation of the adaptive thermogenesis response, an evolutionary mechanism that has greatly expanded the footprint of mammalians on a wide range of climates. The ability to promote substrate utilization has the obvious appeal of an "effortless diet pill," but the capacity of the system is probably insufficient to generate alone a negative energy balance to induce weight loss. Nonetheless, even a modest increase in substrate utilization has been proven able to positively impact energy and carbohydrate metabolism. Thus, the search for novel pharmacologic interventions able to expand the beige adipocytes mass, and thereby increase the capacity for non-shivering thermogenesis, holds the promise of being a successful treatment to improve insulin resistance and the negative metabolic consequences of obesity.

References

Agrawal A, Nair N, Baghel NS (2009) A novel approach for reduction of brown fat uptake on FDG PET. Br J Radiol 82:626–631

Bostrom P, Wu J, Jedrychowski MP, Korde A, Ye L, Lo JC, Rasbach KA, Bostrom EA, Choi JH, Long JZ, Kajimura S, Zingaretti MC, Vind BF, Tu H, Cinti S, Hojlund K, Gygi SP, Spiegelman

BM (2012) A PGC1-alpha-dependent myokine that drives brown-fat-like development of white fat and thermogenesis. Nature 481:463–468

Celi FS (2009) Brown adipose tissue—when it pays to be inefficient. N Engl J Med 360:1553–1556

Celi FS, Brychta RJ, Linderman JD, Butler PW, Alberobello AT, Smith S, Courville AB, Lai EW, Costello R, Skarulis MC, Csako G, Remaley A, Pacak K, Chen KY (2010) Minimal changes in environmental temperature result in a significant increase in energy expenditure and changes in the hormonal homeostasis in healthy adults. Eur J Endocrinol 163:863–872

Celi FS, Le TN, Ni B (2015) Physiology and relevance of human adaptive thermogenesis response. Trends Endocrinol Metab 26:238–247

Chen KY, Brychta RJ, Linderman JD, Smith S, Courville A, Dieckmann W, Herscovitch P, Millo CM, Remaley A, Lee P, Celi FS (2013) Brown fat activation mediates cold-induced thermogenesis in adult humans in response to a mild decrease in ambient temperature. J Clin Endocrinol Metab 98:E1218–E1223

Cypess AM, Lehman S, Williams G, Tal I, Rodman D, Goldfine AB, Kuo FC, Palmer EL, Tseng YH, Doria A, Kolodny GM, Kahn CR (2009) Identification and importance of brown adipose tissue in adult humans. N Engl J Med 360:1509–1517

Davis TR (1961) Chamber cold acclimatization in man. J Appl Physiol 16:1011–1015

Diaz MB, Herzig S, Vegiopoulos A (2014) Thermogenic adipocytes: from cells to physiology and medicine. Metabolism 63:1238–1249

Drubach LA, Palmer EL 3rd, Connolly LP, Baker A, Zurakowski D, Cypess AM (2011) Pediatric brown adipose tissue: detection, epidemiology, and differences from adults. J Pediatr 159:939–944

Hany TF, Gharehpapagh E, Kamel EM, Buck A, Himms-Hagen J, von Schulthess GK (2002) Brown adipose tissue: a factor to consider in symmetrical tracer uptake in the neck and upper chest region. Eur J Nucl Med Mol Imaging 29:1393–1398

Huttunen P, Hirvonen J, Kinnula V (1981) The occurrence of brown adipose tissue in outdoor workers. Eur J Appl Physiol Occup Physiol 46:339–345

Ishibashi J, Seale P (2010) Medicine. Beige can be slimming. Science 328:1113–1114

Kharitonenkov A, Adams AC (2014) Inventing new medicines: the FGF21 story. Mol Metab 3:221–229

Lee P, Brychta RJ, Linderman J, Smith S, Chen KY, Celi FS (2013) Mild cold exposure modulates fibroblast growth factor 21 (FGF21) diurnal rhythm in humans: relationship between FGF21 levels, lipolysis, and cold-induced thermogenesis. J Clin Endocrinol Metab 98:E98–102

Lee P, Werner CD, Kebebew E, Celi FS (2014a) Functional thermogenic beige adipogenesis is inducible in human neck fat. Int J Obes (Lond) 38:170–176

Lee P, Smith S, Linderman J, Courville AB, Brychta RJ, Dieckmann W, Werner CD, Chen KY, Celi FS (2014b) Temperature-acclimated brown adipose tissue modulates insulin sensitivity in humans. Diabetes 63:3686–3698

Lee P, Linderman JD, Smith S, Brychta RJ, Wang J, Idelson C, Perron RM, Werner CD, Phan GQ, Kammula US, Kebebew E, Pacak K, Chen KY, Celi FS (2014c) Irisin and FGF21 are cold-induced endocrine activators of brown fat function in humans. Cell Metab 19:302–309

Nedergaard J, Golozoubova V, Matthias A, Asadi A, Jacobsson A, Cannon B (2001) UCP1: the only protein able to mediate adaptive non-shivering thermogenesis and metabolic inefficiency. Biochim Biophys Acta 1504:82–106

Ni B, Farrar JS, Vaitkus JA, Celi FS (2015) Metabolic effects of FGF-21: thermoregulation and beyond. Front Endocrinol (Lausanne) 6:148

Petrovic N, Walden TB, Shabalina IG, Timmons JA, Cannon B, Nedergaard J (2010) Chronic peroxisome proliferator-activated receptor gamma (PPARgamma) activation of epididymally derived white adipocyte cultures reveals a population of thermogenically competent, UCP1-containing adipocytes molecularly distinct from classic brown adipocytes. J Biol Chem 285:7153–7164

Pfannenberg C, Werner MK, Ripkens S, Stef I, Deckert A, Schmadl M, Reimold M, Haring HU, Claussen CD, Stefan N (2010) Impact of age on the relationships of brown adipose tissue with sex and adiposity in humans. Diabetes 59:1789–1793

Phillips PK, Heath JE (1995) Dependency of surface temperature regulation on body size in terrestrial mammals. J Therm Biol 20:281–289

Ravussin E, Galgani JE (2011) The implication of brown adipose tissue for humans. Annu Rev Nutr 31:33–47

Ravussin Y, Xiao C, Gavrilova O, Reitman ML (2014) Effect of intermittent cold exposure on brown fat activation, obesity, and energy homeostasis in mice. PLoS One 9:e85876

Saito M, Okamatsu-Ogura Y, Matsushita M, Watanabe K, Yoneshiro T, Nio-Kobayashi J, Iwanaga T, Miyagawa M, Kameya T, Nakada K, Kawai Y, Tsujisaki M (2009) High incidence of metabolically active brown adipose tissue in healthy adult humans: effects of cold exposure and adiposity. Diabetes 58:1526–1531

Seale P, Bjork B, Yang W, Kajimura S, Chin S, Kuang S, Scime A, Devarakonda S, Conroe HM, Erdjument-Bromage H, Tempst P, Rudnicki MA, Beier DR, Spiegelman BM (2008) PRDM16 controls a brown fat/skeletal muscle switch. Nature 454:961–967

Shinoda K, Luijten IH, Hasegawa Y, Hong H, Sonne SB, Kim M, Xue R, Chondronikola M, Cypess AM, Tseng YH, Nedergaard J, Sidossis LS, Kajimura S (2015) Genetic and functional characterization of clonally derived adult human brown adipocytes. Nat Med 21:389–394

Stocks JM, Taylor NA, Tipton MJ, Greenleaf JE (2004) Human physiological responses to cold exposure. Aviat Space Environ Med 75:444–457

van der Lans AA, Hoeks J, Brans B, Vijgen GH, Visser MG, Vosselman MJ, Hansen J, Jorgensen JA, Wu J, Mottaghy FM, Schrauwen P, van Marken Lichtenbelt WD (2013) Cold acclimation recruits human brown fat and increases nonshivering thermogenesis. J Clin Invest 123:3395–3403

van Marken Lichtenbelt WD, Vanhommerig JW, Smulders NM, Drossaerts JM, Kemerink GJ, Bouvy ND, Schrauwen P, Teule GJ (2009) Cold-activated brown adipose tissue in healthy men. N Engl J Med 360:1500–1508

Vianna CR, Hagen T, Zhang CY, Bachman E, Boss O, Gereben B, Moriscot AS, Lowell BB, Bicudo JE, Bianco AC (2001) Cloning and functional characterization of an uncoupling protein homolog in hummingbirds. Physiol Genomics 5:137–145

Virtanen KA, Lidell ME, Orava J, Heglind M, Westergren R, Niemi T, Taittonen M, Laine J, Savisto NJ, Enerback S, Nuutila P (2009) Functional brown adipose tissue in healthy adults. N Engl J Med 360:1518–1525

Yoneshiro T, Aita S, Matsushita M, Kameya T, Nakada K, Kawai Y, Saito M (2011) Brown adipose tissue, whole-body energy expenditure, and thermogenesis in healthy adult men. Obesity (Silver Spring) 19:13–16

Yoneshiro T, Aita S, Matsushita M, Kayahara T, Kameya T, Kawai Y, Iwanaga T, Saito M (2013) Recruited brown adipose tissue as an antiobesity agent in humans. J Clin Invest 123:3404–3408

The Energy Sensor AMPK: Adaptations to Exercise, Nutritional and Hormonal Signals

Check for updates

Benoit Viollet

Abstract To sustain metabolism, intracellular ATP concentration must be regulated within an appropriate range. This coordination is achieved through the function of the AMP-activated protein kinase (AMPK), a cellular "fuel gauge" that is expressed in essentially all eukaryotic cells as heterotrimeric complexes containing catalytic α subunits and regulatory β and γ subunits. When cellular energy status has been compromised, AMPK is activated by increases in AMP:ATP or ADP:ATP ratios and acts to restore energy homeostasis by stimulating energy production via catabolic pathways while decreasing non-essential energy-consuming pathways. Although the primary function of AMPK is to regulate energy homeostasis at a cell-autonomous level, in multicellular organisms, the AMPK system has evolved to interact with hormones to regulate energy intake and expenditure at the whole body level. Thus, AMPK functions as a signaling hub, coordinating anabolic and catabolic pathways to balance nutrient supply with energy demand at both the cellular and whole-body levels. AMPK is activated by various metabolic stresses such as ischemia or hypoxia or glucose deprivation and has both acute and long-term effects on metabolic pathways and key cellular functions. In addition, AMPK appears to be a major sensor of energy demand in exercising muscle and acts both as a multitask gatekeeper and an energy regulator in skeletal muscle. Acute activation of AMPK has been shown to promote glucose transport and fatty acid oxidation while suppressing glycogen synthase activity and protein synthesis. Chronic activation of AMPK induces a shift in muscle fiber type composition, reduces markers of muscle degeneration and enhances muscle oxidative capacity potentially by stimulating mitochondrial biogenesis. Furthermore, recent evidence demonstrates that AMPK may not only regulate metabolism during exercise but also in the recovery phase. AMPK acts as a molecular transducer between exercise and insulin signaling and is

B. Viollet (✉)
Institut Cochin, INSERM, U1016, Paris, France

CNRS, UMR8104, Paris, France

Université Paris Descartes, Sorbonne Paris cité, Paris, France
e-mail: benoit.viollet@inserm.fr

© The Author(s) 2017
B. Spiegelman (ed.), *Hormones, Metabolism and the Benefits of Exercise*,
Research and Perspectives in Endocrine Interactions,
https://doi.org/10.1007/978-3-319-72790-5_2

13

necessary for the ability of prior contraction/exercise to increase muscle insulin sensitivity. Based on these observations, drugs that activate AMPK might be expected to be useful in the treatment of metabolic disorders and insulin resistance in various conditions.

Introduction

One fundamental parameter that living cells need to sustain essential cellular functions is the maintenance of sufficiently high level of ATP. Thus, cell survival is dependent on a dynamic control of energy metabolism when ATP demand needs to remain in balance with ATP supply. If ATP consumption exceeds ATP production, the ADP:ATP ratio rises, but this is converted into an even larger rise in AMP:ATP ratio due to the reaction catalyzed by adenylate kinase ($2ADP \leftrightarrow ATP + AMP$). If the reaction is at equilibrium, the AMP:ATP ratio will vary as the square of the ADP:ATP ratio, making increases in AMP a more sensitive indicator of energy stress than decreases in ATP or increases in ADP. On this basis, the cell requires an efficient energy sensory mechanism based on the detection of the ratios of ADP:ATP or AMP:ATP. Such a system has been identified as the AMP-activated protein kinase (AMPK), a heterotrimeric serine/threonine kinase conserved throughout eukaryote evolution (Hardie et al. 2012). The primary function of AMPK is to monitor changes in the intracellular level of ATP and maintain energy stores by reprogramming metabolism through an increase in the rate of catabolic ATP-producing pathways and a decrease in the rate of nonessential anabolic ATP-utilizing pathways. These regulatory features are initiated by the phosphorylation of key metabolic enzyme as well as transcription factors for both short-term effects and long-range regulatory actions for a better response to future challenges. Although the AMPK system originally evolved to regulate energy homeostasis in a cell-autonomous manner, in multicellular organisms, its role has adapted to integrate stress responses such as exercise as well as nutrient and hormonal signals to control food intake, energy expenditure, and substrate utilization at the whole body level (Hardie 2014). Activation of AMPK is triggered by a diverse array of external (e.g., exercise, hormones, nutrients) and internal signals (e.g., AMP/ATP and ADP/ATP ratios) and has been implicated in the regulation of a wide range of biochemical pathways and physiological processes. As a consequence, AMPK has stimulated much interest due to its potential impact on metabolic disorders. The aim of this chapter is to discuss the possible role of AMPK in the adaptations to exercise, nutrient and hormonal signals and its potential as a therapeutic drug target, mimicking the beneficial effects of exercise.

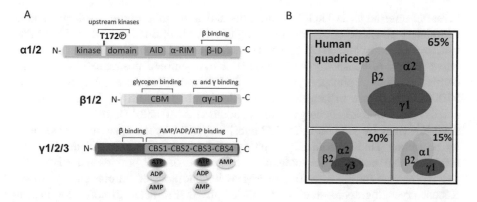

Fig. 1 Schematic representation of AMPK subunit. (**a**) AMPK domain structure. (**b**) AMPK heterotrimer composition in human skeletal muscle

AMPK: Structure and Regulation

AMPK is a heterotrimeric complex composed of one catalytic α-subunit comprising a typical Ser/Thr kinase domain, in combination with scaffolding β-subunit containing a carbohydrate binding module (CBM) and γ-subunit containing four cystathionine-β-synthase (CBS) domains that serve to bind adenine nucleotides (Fig. 1). Each of these subunits has several isoforms encoded by different genes (α1, α2, β1, β2, γ1, γ2 and γ3) that can theoretically combine to form 12 possible heterotrimeric complexes (Hardie et al. 2012). Differential expression of the AMPK isoform in tissues and post-translational modifications that may locate AMPK in different cellular compartments also contribute to the specialized functions of AMPK heterotrimeric complexes. Of interest, in contrast to other AMPK isoforms, expression of the AMPKγ3 isoform is restricted to the fast-twitch glycolytic skeletal muscle, suggesting a particular role for AMPKγ3-containing complexes to handle metabolic challenges in skeletal muscle (Barnes et al. 2004). Mutation in the gene encoding for the AMPKγ3 subunit PRKAG3 has been reported in pigs and humans, causing increased deposition of glycogen in skeletal muscle (Milan et al. 2000; Costford et al. 2007). In human skeletal muscle, only three heterotrimeric complexes have been detected, α2β2γ1 (65% of the total pool), α2β2γ3 (20%), and α1β2γ1 (15%) (Birk and Wojtaszewski 2006; Fig. 1). The heterotrimer combination varies in mouse skeletal muscle, with the detection of five complexes, including α1 and α2-associated AMPK complexes with both β1 and β2 isoforms (Treebak et al. 2009). Interestingly, each heterotrimer combination displays a distinct activation profile in response to physical exercise, with γ3-containing complexes being predominantly activated and α2β2γ1 and α1β2γ1 heterotrimers being unchanged or activated only after prolonged exercise (Birk and Wojtaszewski 2006).

The mechanism of AMPK activation involves two steps, a reversible phosphorylation at a conserved residue (Thr174 in α1 and Thr172 in α2 catalytic subunit, hereafter referred to as Thr172) within the activation loop in the α-subunit, and a stimulatory allosteric effect upon binding of AMP within the CBS domains of the γ-subunit (Hardie et al. 2012). Activity of the complex increases more than 100-fold when AMPK is phosphorylated on Thr172 by identified upstream kinases. The combined effect of phosphorylation on Thr172 and allosteric regulation causes a >1000-fold increase in kinase activity, allowing high sensitivity in responses to small changes in cellular energy status. In addition, AMP and ADP binding regulates AMPK activity by promoting Thr172 phosphorylation by the upstream kinases and by protecting Thr172 from dephosphorylation by phosphatases. All the binding effects of AMP and ADP are antagonized by binding of ATP, providing a very sensitive mechanism for the activation of AMPK in conditions of cellular energy stress. Recent crystallographic studies of full-length AMPK heterotrimeric complexes have provided insights into the domain structure and the regulation upon binding of adenosine nucleotides (Hardie et al. 2016). Because the activating ligand is bound on the γ subunit and the kinase domain is in the α subunit, intersubunit communication has to occur when switching to fully active states. Important regulatory features for this conformational switch are provided by α subunit flexible components (Fig. 1), the autoinhibitory domain (AID) and the α-regulatory subunit interacting motif (α-RIM)/α-hook interacting with the exchangeable nucleotide-binding sites on the γ subunit, offering a signaling mechanism for nucleotide allosteric regulation and protection against dephosphorylation of AMPK heterotrimeric complex.

In mammals, the major upstream kinases are the liver kinase B1 (LKB1) and Ca2+/calmodulin-dependent protein kinase kinase 2 (CaMKK2; Hardie et al. 2012). Interestingly, CaMKK2 has been shown to phosphorylate and activate AMPK in response to an increase in intracellular Ca^{2+} concentration, independent of any change in cellular AMP:ATP or ADP:ATP ratios. In skeletal muscle, the major upstream kinase phosphorylating α subunit Thr172 is liver kinase B1 (LKB1), as exercise-induced AMPK phosphorylation is prevented in mouse models lacking LKB1 (Sakamoto et al. 2005; Thomson et al. 2007). However, CaMKKβ has been shown to activate AMPK during mild tetanic skeletal muscle contraction (Jensen et al. 2007) and to increase AMPKα1 activity in response to skeletal muscle overload in LKB1-deficient mice (McGee et al. 2008).

AMPK: Regulation by Hormones and Nutrients

Although AMPK was originally identified as a sensor of cellular energy status by coordinating anabolic and catabolic pathways to balance nutrient supply with energy demand, it is now clear that it also participates in controlling whole-body energy homeostasis by integrating hormonal and nutritional signals from the cellular environment and the whole organism. Hypothalamic AMPK has been suggested to be a key mediator in the regulation of neuronal regulation of feeding behaviour and energy balance (Fig. 2). Inhibition of AMPK by expressing a dominant negative isoform in the arcuate nucleus (ARC) of the hypothalamus decreases mRNA

Fig. 2 Hypothalamic AMPK in the regulation of energy balance

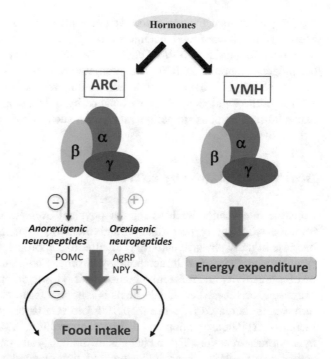

expression of the orexigenic neuropeptides agouti-related peptide (AgRP) and neu-ropeptide Y (NPY; Minokoshi et al. 2004). Conversely, activation of AMPK in the ARC by expressing a constitutively active AMPK form can further increase the fasting-induced expression of AgRP and NPY and then elevated feeding (Minokoshi et al. 2004). Similarly, starvation induces AMPK activation and food intake. In con-trast, refeeding and glucose administration promote AMPK inactivation, accompa-nied by increased levels of anorexigenic neuropeptides proopiomelanocortin (POMC) and reduced levels of orexigenic neuropeptides AgRP mRNA in the ARC, highlighting the sensing levels of nutrients in the hypothalamus (Andersson et al. 2004; Minokoshi et al. 2004). There are also a number of hormones involved in the regulation of appetite that alter AMPK activity in the hypothalamus. For example, the orexigenic hormones, such as ghrelin and adiponectin, activate AMPK in the ARC and promote food intake (Andersson et al. 2004; Kubota et al. 2007); in con-trast, anorectic hormones, such as leptin and oestradiol, inhibit AMPK in the ARC and inhibit food intake (Yang et al. 2011; Martinez de Morentin et al. 2014). Another layer of signal integration for the regulation of whole-body energy balance happens at the level of the ventromedial nucleus (VMH) of the hypothalamus, where AMPK regulates energy expenditure by controlling brown adipose tissue (BAT) thermogen-esis (López et al. 2010; Whittle et al. 2012; Beiroa et al. 2014; Martinez de Morentin et al. 2014). Importantly, expression of a constitutively active AMPK form in the VMH is associated with a specific reduction in the expression of BAT thermogenic markers. In contrast, inhibition of AMPK by administration of thyroid hormone T3 to the VMH promotes whole body energy expenditure by triggering BAT thermogenesis via activation of the sympathetic nervous system (López et al. 2010). More recently, it was found that injection of glucagon-like peptide-1 (GLP-1) receptor agonist liraglutide into VMH decreased AMPK activity, stimulated expression of thermogenic markers in BAT, and promoted weight loss without affecting food intake (Beiroa et al. 2014). Overall these findings demonstrate a key role for central AMPK in the regulation of energy balance by influencing food intake and energy expenditure in response to peripheral signals, such as hormones and nutrients.

AMPK: Regulation by Exercise

Lifestyle intervention such as regular physical exercise is widely recognized to improve whole-body performance and metabolism in health and disease. An increase in daily physical activity is an effective approach to combat many disease symptoms associated with metabolic syndrome. Endurance exercise can improve insulin sensitivity and metabolic homeostasis. However, our understanding of how exercise exerts these beneficial effects is incomplete. In response to exercise, ATP turnover is increased by more than 100-fold (Gaitanos et al. 1993), resulting in increased ATP consumption and a rise in intracellular AMP levels due to the adenylate kinase reaction. These changes in the adenylate energy charge lead to the activation of AMPK in an intensity- and time-dependent manner, as shown in rodents (Winder and Hardie 1996) and in human muscle (Wojtaszewski et al. 2000). Once activated, AMPK regulates multiple signaling pathways whose overall effects are to increase ATP production, including fatty acid oxidation and glucose uptake. Given that AMPK is at the nexus of metabolic signaling pathways, a great deal of interest has focused on the role of AMPK in the adaptation of skeletal muscle to exercise as well as its use as a possible therapeutic target for the treatment of type 2 diabetes.

Control of Exercise-Induced Glucose Transport

During exercise, contracting skeletal muscle rapidly increases glucose uptake in an intensity-dependent manner to sustain the energy demand caused by increased ATP turnover. The first compelling evidence for a role for AMPK in regulating glucose uptake in skeletal muscle has been obtained with pharmacological activation of AMPK by AICAR (Merrill et al. 1997). This finding was further supported by the observation of impaired response to AICAR stimulation in mice expressing a dominant negative AMPK form in skeletal muscle (Mu et al. 2001). However, the role for AMPK in regulating glucose uptake during muscle contractile activity remains controversial and no solid genetic evidence has been put forward. Exercise-induced muscle glucose uptake is impaired in AMPK β1β2M-KO mice but remains intact in AMPKα mdKO (O'Neill et al. 2011; Lantier et al. 2014). The reason for the

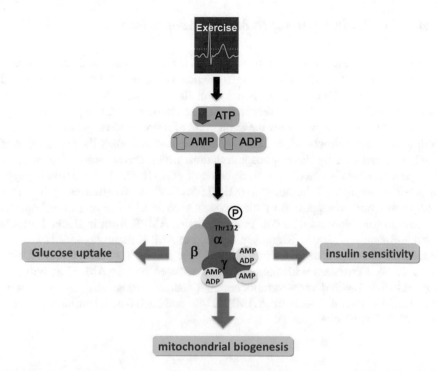

Fig. 3 AMPK-mediated regulation of skeletal muscle adaptation to exercise

difference between studies is not clear and future studies using inducible mouse models to study the role of AMPK in developed adult skeletal muscle are warranted.

It has been suggested that AMPK enhances glucose uptake by increasing the translocation of glucose transporter type 4 (GLUT4) to the plasma membrane (Fig. 3). Recent findings using AMPK-deficient mouse models have shown a convergence to the phosphorylation of the downstream target of TBC1D1, Rab-GTPase activating protein, which is emerging as an essential player in contraction-stimulated GLUT4 translocation (Stockli et al. 2015). In support of this finding, mice expressing TBC1D1 that mutated at predicted AMPK phosphorylation sites showed reduced contraction-stimulated glucose uptake (Vichaiwong et al. 2010). Interestingly, in exercised human skeletal muscle, TBC1D1 phosphorylation was significantly correlated with the activity of the $\alpha2\beta2\gamma3$ heterotrimer, supporting the idea that AMPK is a direct upstream TBC1D1 kinase (Treebak et al. 2014).

Recent studies using compound 991, a cyclic benzimidazole derivative and potent direct AMPK activator, have shown that pharmacological activation of AMPK is sufficient to elicit metabolic effects in muscle appropriate for treating type 2 diabetes (Lai et al. 2014). It is also important to note that AMPK-mediated glucose uptake is not impaired in type 2 diabetes during exercise (Musi et al. 2001); therefore, activation of AMPK represents an attractive target for intervention.

Control of Training-Induced Muscle Adaptations

In response to repeated metabolic stress, AMPK orchestrates a coordinated response to enhance mitochondrial biogenesis to match substrate utilization to demand (Fig. 3; Zong et al. 2002). This response is mediated through the regulation of peroxisome proliferator-activated receptor γ co-activator-1α (PGC-1α), a transcriptional co-activator that promotes the expression of mitochondrial genes encoded in both nuclear and mitochondrial DNA. AMPK activation causes the stimulation of PGC-1α expression by direct phosphorylation, which drives expression from its own promoter but also involves deacetylation of PGC-1α via the silent mating-type information regulator 2 homolog 1 (SIRT1; McGee and Hargreaves 2010). This finding was further supported by the increase seen in PGC-1α and mitochondrial function in mice expressing a constitutively active AMPK form in skeletal muscle (Garcia-Roves et al. 2008). Moreover, deletion of AMPK greatly reduced exercise-induced SIRT1-dependent activation of PGC-1α signaling in skeletal muscle (Canto et al. 2010). Consistent with these findings, reduced muscle AMPK activity has been associated with decreased mitochondrial content during aging (Reznick et al. 2007) and in skeletal muscle from AMPKβ1β2- and LKB1-deficient mice (O'Neill et al. 2011; Tanner et al. 2013).

Control of Muscle Insulin Sensitivity

Skeletal muscle demonstrates increased insulin-stimulated glucose uptake in the period after exercise (Richter et al. 1982). It may involve an increased translocation of GLUT4 at the plasma membrane in response to insulin. The underlying mechanism appears to involve AMPK-dependent phosphorylation of the Rab-GTPase TBC1D4 regulating GLUT4 translocation (Kjobsted et al. 2016). These results are fully in line with previous findings showing that prior pharmacological AMPK activation by AICAR enhances insulin sensitivity in rat skeletal muscle with increased phosphorylation of TBC1D4 (Kjobsted et al. 2015). Thus, activation of AMPK in the recovery after exercise may be important for exercise-induced adaptations and may serve to enhance muscle insulin sensitivity (Fig. 3). These findings may be highly relevant for pharmacological interventions in the treatment of muscle insulin resistance.

Conclusions and Therapeutic Perspectives

In mammals, AMPK has emerged as a major energy sensor that integrates multiple extracellular and intracellular input signals to coordinate cellular energy balance. Targeted by nutritional and hormone signals, AMPK has a crucial role in the hypothalamus to regulate energy intake and energy expenditure. In skeletal muscle, AMPK has been identified as an important integrator of the metabolic changes that occur during physical exercise. Given these roles, AMPK is an obvious target for treatment of metabolic disorders such as obesity and diabetes. However, although pharmacological activation in peripheral organs is expected to provide therapeutic benefits, activating central AMPK could cause deleterious consequences, specifically on body weight control. Recent studies have highlighted the adverse metabolic consequence of AMPK activation throughout all tissues (Yavari et al. 2016). Thus, a better understanding of the precise role of AMPK in the cell and its effects at the whole-body level will be essential for delineating therapeutic strategies aimed at targeting AMPK.

References

Andersson U, Filipsson K, Abbott CR, Woods A, Smith K, Bloom SR, Carling D, Small CJ (2004) AMP-activated protein kinase plays a role in the control of food intake. J Biol Chem 279:12005–12008

Barnes BR, Marklund S, Steiler TL, Walter M, Hjalm G, Amarger V, Mahlapuu M, Leng Y, Johansson C, Galuska D, Lindgren K, Abrink M, Stapleton D, Zierath JR, Andersson L (2004) The 5′-AMP-activated protein kinase gamma3 isoform has a key role in carbohydrate and lipid metabolism in glycolytic skeletal muscle. J Biol Chem 279:38441–38447

Beiroa D, Imbernon M, Gallego R, Senra A, Herranz D, Villarroya F, Serrano M, Ferno J, Salvador J, Escalada J, Dieguez C, Lopez M, Fruhbeck G, Nogueiras R (2014) GLP-1 agonism stimulates brown adipose tissue thermogenesis and browning through hypothalamic AMPK. Diabetes 63:3346–3358

Birk JB, Wojtaszewski JF (2006) Predominant alpha2/beta2/gamma3 AMPK activation during exercise in human skeletal muscle. J Physiol 577:1021–1032

Canto C, Jiang LQ, Deshmukh AS, Mataki C, Coste A, Lagouge M, Zierath JR, Auwerx J (2010) Interdependence of AMPK and SIRT1 for metabolic adaptation to fasting and exercise in skeletal muscle. Cell Metab 11:213–219

Costford SR, Kavaslar N, Ahituv N, Chaudhry SN, Schackwitz WS, Dent R, Pennacchio LA, McPherson R, Harper ME (2007) Gain-of-function R225W mutation in human AMPKgamma(3) causing increased glycogen and decreased triglyceride in skeletal muscle. PLoS One 2:e903

Gaitanos GC, Williams C, Boobis LH, Brooks S (1993) Human muscle metabolism during intermittent maximal exercise. J Appl Physiol (1985) 75:712–719

Garcia Roves PM, Osler ME, Holmstrom MH, Zierath JR (2008) Gain-of-function R225Q mutation in AMP-activated protein kinase gamma3 subunit increases mitochondrial biogenesis in glycolytic skeletal muscle. J Biol Chem 283:35724–35734

Hardie DG (2014) AMPK-sensing energy while talking to other signaling pathways. Cell Metab 20:939–952

Hardie DG, Ross FA, Hawley SA (2012) AMPK: a nutrient and energy sensor that maintains energy homeostasis. Nat Rev Mol Cell Biol 13:251–262

Hardie DG, Schaffer BE, Brunet A (2016) AMPK: An energy-sensing pathway with multiple inputs and outputs. Trends Cell Biol 26:190–201

Jensen TE, Rose AJ, Jorgensen SB, Brandt N, Schjerling P, Wojtaszewski JF, Richter EA (2007) Possible CaMKK-dependent regulation of AMPK phosphorylation and glucose uptake at the onset of mild tetanic skeletal muscle contraction. Am J Physiol Endocrinol Metab 292:E1308–E1317

Kjobsted R, Treebak JT, Fentz J, Lantier L, Viollet B, Birk JB, Schjerling P, Bjornholm M, Zierath JR, Wojtaszewski JF (2015) Prior AICAR stimulation increases insulin sensitivity in mouse skeletal muscle in an AMPK-dependent manner. Diabetes 64:2042–2055

Kjobsted R, Munk-Hansen N, Birk JB, Foretz M, Viollet B, Bjornholm M, Zierath JR, Treebak JT, Wojtaszewski JF (2016) Enhanced muscle insulin sensitivity after contraction/exercise is mediated by AMPK. Diabetes. pii: db160530

Kubota N, Yano W, Kubota T, Yamauchi T, Itoh S, Kumagai H, Kozono H, Takamoto I, Okamoto S, Shiuchi T, Suzuki R, Satoh H, Tsuchida A, Moroi M, Sugi K, Noda T, Ebinuma H, Ueta Y, Kondo T, Araki E, Ezaki O, Nagai R, Tobe K, Terauchi Y, Ueki K, Minokoshi Y, Kadowaki T (2007) Adiponectin stimulates AMP-activated protein kinase in the hypothalamus and increases food intake. Cell Metab 6:55–68

Lai YC, Kviklyte S, Vertommen D, Lantier L, Foretz M, Viollet B, Hallen S, Rider MH (2014) A small-molecule benzimidazole derivative that potently activates AMPK to increase glucose transport in skeletal muscle: comparison with effects of contraction and other AMPK activators. Biochem J 460:363–375

Lantier L, Fentz J, Mounier R, Leclerc J, Treebak JT, Pehmoller C, Sanz N, Sakakibara I, Saint-Amand E, Rimbaud S, Maire P, Marette A, Ventura-Clapier R, Ferry A, Wojtaszewski JF, Foretz M, Viollet B (2014) AMPK controls exercise endurance, mitochondrial oxidative capacity, and skeletal muscle integrity. FASEB J 28:3211–3224

López M, Varela L, Vázquez MJ, Rodríguez-Cuenca S, González CR, Velagapudi VR, Morgan DA, Schoenmakers E, Agassandian K, Lage R, Martínez de Morentin PB, Tovar S, Nogueiras R, Carling D, Lelliott C, Gallego R, Oresic M, Chatterjee K, Saha AK, Rahmouni K, Diéguez C, Vidal-Puig A (2010) Hypothalamic AMPK and fatty acid metabolism mediate thyroid regulation of energy balance. Nat Med 16:1001–1008

Martinez de Morentin PB, Gonzalez-Garcia I, Martins L, Lage R, Fernandez-Mallo D, Martinez-Sanchez N, Ruiz-Pino F, Liu J, Morgan DA, Pinilla L, Gallego R, Saha AK, Kalsbeek A, Fliers E, Bisschop PH, Dieguez C, Nogueiras R, Rahmouni K, Tena-Sempere M, Lopez M (2014) Estradiol regulates brown adipose tissue thermogenesis via hypothalamic AMPK. Cell Metab 20:41–53

McGee SL, Hargreaves M (2010) AMPK-mediated regulation of transcription in skeletal muscle. Clin Sci (Lond) 118:507–518

McGee SL, Mustard KJ, Hardie DG, Baar K (2008) Normal hypertrophy accompanied by phosphoryation and activation of AMP-activated protein kinase alpha1 following overload in LKB1 knockout mice. J Physiol 586:1731–1741

Merrill GF, Kurth EJ, Hardie DG, Winder WW (1997) AICA riboside increases AMP-activated protein kinase, fatty acid oxidation, and glucose uptake in rat muscle. Am J Physiol 273:E1107–E1112

Milan D, Jeon JT, Looft C, Amarger V, Robic A, Thelander M, Rogel-Gaillard C, Paul S, Iannuccelli N, Rask L, Ronne H, Lundstrom K, Reinsch N, Gellin J, Kalm E, Roy PL, Chardon P, Andersson L (2000) A mutation in PRKAG3 associated with excess glycogen content in pig skeletal muscle. Science 288:1248–1251

Minokoshi Y, Alquier T, Furukawa N, Kim YB, Lee A, Xue B, Mu J, Foufelle F, Ferre P, Birnbaum MJ, Stuck BJ, Kahn BB (2004) AMP-kinase regulates food intake by responding to hormonal and nutrient signals in the hypothalamus. Nature 428:569–574

Mu J, Brozinick JT Jr, Valladares O, Bucan M, Birnbaum MJ (2001) A role for AMP-activated protein kinase in contraction- and hypoxia-regulated glucose transport in skeletal muscle. Mol Cell 7:1085–1094

Musi N, Fujii N, Hirshman MF, Ekberg I, Froberg S, Ljungqvist O, Thorell A, Goodyear LJ (2001) AMP-activated protein kinase (AMPK) is activated in muscle of subjects with type 2 diabetes during exercise. Diabetes 50:921–927

O'Neill HM, Maarbjerg SJ, Crane JD, Jeppesen J, Jorgensen SB, Schertzer JD, Shyroka O, Kiens B, van Denderen BJ, Tarnopolsky MA, Kemp BE, Richter EA, Steinberg GR (2011) AMP-activated protein kinase (AMPK) beta1beta2 muscle null mice reveal an essential role for AMPK in maintaining mitochondrial content and glucose uptake during exercise. Proc Natl Acad Sci USA 108:16092–16097

Reznick RM, Zong H, Li J, Morino K, Moore IK, HJ Y, Liu ZX, Dong J, Mustard KJ, Hawley SA, Befroy D, Pypaert M, Hardie DG, Young LH, Shulman GI (2007) Aging-associated reductions in AMP-activated protein kinase activity and mitochondrial biogenesis. Cell Metab 5:151–156

Richter EA, Garetto LP, Goodman MN, Ruderman NB (1982) Muscle glucose metabolism following exercise in the rat: increased sensitivity to insulin. J Clin Invest 69:785–793

Sakamoto K, McCarthy A, Smith D, Green KA, Grahame Hardie D, Ashworth A, Alessi DR (2005) Deficiency of LKB1 in skeletal muscle prevents AMPK activation and glucose uptake during contraction. EMBO J 24:1810–1820

Stockli J, Meoli CC, Hoffman NJ, Fazakerley DJ, Pant H, Cleasby ME, Ma X, Kleinert M, Brandon AE, Lopez JA, Cooney GJ, James DE (2015) The RabGAP TBC1D1 plays a central role in exercise-regulated glucose metabolism in skeletal muscle. Diabetes 64:1914–1922

Tanner CB, Madsen SR, Hallowell DM, Goring DM, Moore TM, Hardman SE, Heninger MR, Atwood DR, Thomson DM (2013) Mitochondrial and performance adaptations to exercise training in mice lacking skeletal muscle LKB1. Am J Physiol Endocrinol Metab 305:E1018–E1029

Thomson DM, Porter BB, Tall JH, Kim HJ, Barrow JR, Winder WW (2007) Skeletal muscle and heart LKB1 deficiency causes decreased voluntary running and reduced muscle mitochondrial marker enzyme expression in mice. Am J Physiol Endocrinol Metab 292:E196–E202

Treebak JT, Birk JB, Hansen BF, Olsen GS, Wojtaszewski JF (2009) A-769662 activates AMPK beta1-containing complexes but induces glucose uptake through a PI3-kinase-dependent pathway in mouse skeletal muscle. Am J Physiol Cell Physiol 297:C1041–C1052

Treebak JT, Pehmoller C, Kristensen JM, Kjobsted R, Birk JB, Schjerling P, Richter EA, Goodyear LJ, Wojtaszewski JF (2014) Acute exercise and physiological insulin induce distinct phosphorylation signatures on TBC1D1 and TBC1D4 proteins in human skeletal muscle. J Physiol 592:351–375

Vichaiwong K, Purohit S, An D, Toyoda T, Jessen N, Hirshman MF, Goodyear LJ (2010) Contraction regulates site-specific phosphorylation of TBC1D1 in skeletal muscle. Biochem J 431:311–320

Whittle AJ, Carobbio S, Martins L, Slawik M, Hondares E, Vazquez MJ, Morgan D, Csikasz RI, Gallego R, Rodriguez-Cuenca S, Dale M, Virtue S, Villarroya F, Cannon B, Rahmouni K, Lopez M, Vidal-Puig A (2012) BMP8B increases brown adipose tissue thermogenesis through both central and peripheral actions. Cell 149:871–885

Winder WW, Hardie DG (1996) Inactivation of acetyl-CoA carboxylase and activation of AMP-activated protein kinase in muscle during exercise. Am J Physiol 270:E299–E304

Wojtaszewski JF, Nielsen P, Hansen BF, Richter EA, Kiens B (2000) Isoform-specific and exercise intensity-dependent activation of 5'-AMP-activated protein kinase in human skeletal muscle. J Physiol 528(Pt 1):221–226

Yang Y, Atasoy D, HH S, Sternson SM (2011) Hunger states switch a flip-flop memory circuit via a synaptic AMPK-dependent positive feedback loop. Cell 146:992–1003

Yavari A, Stocker CJ, Ghaffari S, Wargent ET, Steeples V, Czibik G, Pinter K, Bellahcene M, Woods A, Martínez de Morentin PB, Cansell C, Lam BY, Chuster A, Petkevicius K, Nguyen-Tu MS, Martinez-Sanchez A, Pullen TJ, Oliver PL, Stockenhuber A, Nguyen C, Lazdam M, O'Dowd JF, Harikumar P, Tóth M, Beall C, Kyriakou T, Parnis J, Sarma D, Katritsis G, Wortmann DD, Harper AR, Brown LA, Willows R, Gandra S, Poncio V, de Oliveira Figueiredo MJ, Qi NR, Peirson SN, McCrimmon RJ, Gereben B, Tretter L, Fekete C, Redwood C, Yeo GS, Heisler LK, Rutter GA, Smith MA, Withers DJ, Carling D, Sternick EB, Arch JR, Cawthorne MA,

Watkins H, Ashrafian H (2016) Chronic activation of gamma2 AMPK induces obesity and reduces beta cell function. Cell Metab 23:821–836

Zong H, Ren JM, Young LH, Pypaert M, Mu J, Birnbaum MJ, Shulman GI (2002) AMP kinase is required for mitochondrial biogenesis in skeletal muscle in response to chronic energy deprivation. Proc Natl Acad Sci USA 99:15983–15987

Plasma Steroids and Cardiorespiratory Fitness Response to Regular Exercise

Zihong He, Tuomo Rankinen, Arthur S. Leon, James S. Skinner, André Tchernof, and Claude Bouchard

Abstract The aim of this report is to evaluate the relationships between baseline levels of adrenal, gonadal and conjugated steroids and baseline cardiorespiratory fitness, as assessed by maximal oxygen uptake (VO_2max), as well as its response to a standardized exercise program. To address this aim we used a subset of the HERITAGE Family Study (N = 448). In men, significant positive associations were found between baseline VO_2max/kg weight and plasma levels of androsterone glucuronide (ADTG), dihydrotesterone (DHT), 17 hydroxy progesterone (OHPROG), sex hormone binding globulin (SHBG), and testosterone (TESTO), and negative association with aldosterone (ALDO). In women, only the free androgen index (FAI) was negatively associated with baseline VO_2max/kg weight. Neither baseline plasma steroid levels nor SHBG concentrations were associated with the gains in VO_2max resulting from exposure to the 20-week aerobic exercise program after adjustment for baseline values, age and ethnicity (white or black). We conclude that baseline plasma steroid levels are only weakly associated with individual differences in cardiorespiratory fitness in the sedentary state in men but not in women, whereas no association could be detected with trainability, as defined by the change in VO_2max with the exercise program.

Z. He
Human Genomics Laboratory, Pennington Biomedical Research Center, Baton Rouge, LA, USA

Department of Biology, China Institute of Sport Science, Beijing, China

T. Rankinen • C. Bouchard (✉)
Human Genomics Laboratory, Pennington Biomedical Research Center, Baton Rouge, LA, USA
e-mail: claude.bouchard@pbrc.edu

A. S. Leon
School of Kinesiology, University of Minnesota, Minneapolis, MN, USA

J. S. Skinner
Department of Kinesiology, Indiana University, Bloomington, IN, USA

A. Tchernof
School of Nutrition, Laval University, Quebec City, QC, Canada

© The Author(s) 2017
B. Spiegelman (ed.), *Hormones, Metabolism and the Benefits of Exercise*,
Research and Perspectives in Endocrine Interactions,
https://doi.org/10.1007/978-3-319-72790-5_3

Introduction

The ongoing global epidemic of chronic non-communicable diseases (NCDs) is related to changes in lifestyle, including low physical activity (PA) levels. Physical inactivity is a major public health challenge (Engberg et al. 2012) and has been defined as the fourth leading cause of death worldwide (Kohl et al. 2012). The health benefits of regular PA are well established, and elimination of physical inactivity would remove between 6 and 10% of NCDs and increase life expectancy (Lee et al. 2012). Moreover, cardiorespiratory fitness (CRF) is a strong predictor of health and longevity (United States Department of Health and Human Services 2008). There are large individual differences in CRF among adults who are sedentary and who have a history of not engaging in regular exercise (Bouchard et al. 2015). The response of CRF to regular exercise is also highly variable, even when the exercise prescription is highly standardized and when compliance is not an issue (Skinner et al. 2001). As shown by the findings of the HERITAGE Family Study, there are many factors contributing to variation in CRF exercise training response (Sarzynski et al. 2016). However, little is known about the relationships between plasma levels of steroid hormones and CRF in the sedentary state or in response to regular exercise in men or women.

Steroid hormones are mainly synthesized from cholesterol in the gonads and adrenal glands but some are also produced in other tissues such as skeletal muscle (Sato and Lemitsu 2015), adipose tissue, liver and others (Luu-The and Labrie 2010; Labrie 2015). Steroid hormones can be grouped into two classes, corticosteroids and sex steroids. Within those two classes, there are five types of hormones depending on the receptors to which they bind: glucocorticoids, mineralocorticoids, androgens, estrogens, and progestogens. Steroid hormones are generally carried in the blood, bound to specific carrier proteins such as sex hormone-binding globulin (SHBG; Hammond 2016) or corticosteroid-binding globulin (Meyer et al. 2016).

Steroid hormones exert a wide variety of effects on cardiorespiratory function. In brief, corticosteroids help mediate the stress response and promote energy replenishment and efficient cardiovascular function (Nicolaides et al. 2015). They also regulate muscle function by acting on muscle mass and strength (Hasan et al. 2012). Mineralocorticoids contribute to the regulation of blood pressure and participate in the regulation of cardiac and vascular function. The mineralocorticoid aldosterone (ALDO) is a key regulator of water and electrolyte homeostasis. Clinical trials have shown the beneficial effects of ALDO antagonists in chronic heart failure and post-myocardial infarction treatment (Lother et al. 2015). Long-term infusion of mineralocorticoid (ALDO) in mice resulted in elevation of plasma interleukin-1β levels and vascular abnormalities (Bruder-Nascimento et al. 2016). Androgens enhance skeletal muscle mass by promoting the enlargement of skeletal muscle cells (Sinha-Hikim et al. 2004). Muscle steroid hormone levels were shown to be positively correlated with muscle strength and cross-sectional area (Sato et al. 2014). Also, androgens inhibit the ability of adipocytes to store lipids by blocking a signal transduction pathway (Singh et al. 2006). Androgen deficiency has been shown to be a major risk factor for several disorders, including obesity, metabolic syndrome, and ischemic heart disease (Pongkan et al. 2016). The CARDIA Male Hormone Study showed that there are associations of androgens with PA and fitness in young black and white men (Wolin et al. 2007). Estrogens have vasculo-protective actions that are thought to prevent atherosclerosis (Reslan and Khalil 2012). Estrogens contribute to the regulation of the delicate balance between fighting infections and protecting arteries from damage, thus lowering the risk of cardiovascular disease (Meyer and Barton 2016). Some cardiovascular effects of estrogens may be counteracted by progestogens (Haddock et al. 2000; Group 2006). Progestogens have favorable effects on lipid, glucose and insulin profiles (Group 2006). Higher sex hormone binding globulin (SHBG) concentration was shown to be associated with a more favorable cardiovascular disease (CVD) risk profile, independent of total testosterone (Canoy et al. 2014).

A significant positive correlation has been observed between the changes in serum testosterone levels and the number of steps executed on a daily basis; this finding suggests that the level of PA affects serum testosterone concentrations in overweight and obese men (Kumagai et al. 2016). Steroid hormones are responsive to acute and chronic endurance exercise. Both acute and chronic exercise influence circulating steroid hormone levels (Sato and Lemitsu 2015) and SHBG (Kim and Kim 2012; Ennour-Idrissi et al. 2015) and activate local steroidogenesis in skeletal muscle (Sato and Lemitsu 2015).

In the present report, we focus on the relationships between plasma levels of adrenal, gonadal and conjugated steroids in the sedentary state and baseline (intrinsic) CRF, as assessed by maximal oxygen uptake (VO_2max), as well as its response to a standardized exercise program taking into account factors such as age, gender, ethnicity, and baseline characteristics when appropriate.

Methods

Subjects

The HERITAGE Family Study cohort has been previously described (Bouchard et al. 1995). A total of 488 adults with complete steroid hormones and VO_2max data, who were fully compliant with the 20-week HERITAGE aerobic exercise program, were available for the present study. The study protocol had been previously approved by the institutional review board at each of the four clinical centers of HERITAGE. Informed written consent was obtained from each subject.

Anthropometric and Body Composition Measurements

Body weight and height were measured following standardized procedures. Body density was measured using the hydrostatic weighing technique. The mean of the highest three (of 10) measurements was used in the calculation of percent body fat from body density using the equation of Siri (1956). Fat mass was obtained by multiplying body weight by percent body fat. These measurements have been shown to be highly reproducible, with no difference between clinical centers or drift over time in the course of data collection (Wilmore et al. 1997).

Aerobic Exercise Training Program

Each subject in the HERITAGE study exercised three times per week for 20 weeks on cycle ergometers. The intensity of the training was customized for each individual on the basis of heart rate (HR) and VO_2max measurements taken at a baseline maximal exercise test. Details of the exercise training protocol can be found elsewhere (Bouchard et al. 1995). Briefly, subjects trained at the HR associated with 55% of baseline VO_2max for 30 min per session for the first 2 weeks. The duration and intensity were gradually increased every 2 weeks, until reaching 50 min and 75% of the HR associated with baseline VO_2max. This level was maintained for the final six weeks of training. All training was performed on Universal Aerobicycles (Cedar Rapids, IA) and power output was controlled by direct HR monitoring using the Universal Gym Mednet (Cedar Rapids, IA) computerized system. The protocol was standardized across all four clinical centers and supervised to ensure that the equipment was working properly and that participants were compliant with the protocol.

VO_2max Measurement

Two maximal exercise tests to measure VO_2max were performed on two separate days at baseline and again on two separate days after training using a SensorMedics 800S (Yorba Linda, CA) cycle ergometer and a SensorMedics 2900 metabolic measurement cart (Skinner et al. 2000). The tests were conducted at about the same time of day, with at least 48 h between the two tests. In the first test, subjects exercised at a power output of 50 W for 3 min, followed by increases of 25 W every 2 min until volitional exhaustion. For older, smaller, or less fit individuals, the test was started at 40 W, with increases of 10–20 W every 2 min thereafter. In the second test, subjects exercised for 10 min at an absolute (50 W) and at a relative power output equivalent to 60% VO_2max. They then exercised for 3 min at a relative power output that was 80% of their VO_2max, after which resistance was increased to the highest power output attained in the first maximal test. If the subjects were able to pedal after 2 min, power output was increased every 2 min thereafter until they reached volitional fatigue. The average VO$_2$max from these two sets was taken as the VO$_2$max for that subject and used in analyses if both values were within 5% of each other. If they differed by >5%, the higher VO$_2$max value was used.

Plasma Steroid Hormone and SHBG Concentrations

The hormonal assays have been previously described (Couillard et al. 2000; Ukkola et al. 2001). Fourteen steroid hormones or their derivatives and SHBG concentrations were assayed. Table 1 provides the full name of each hormone, the abbreviations used in the present report and a brief comment on the source of production or

Table 1 Description of steroid hormones assayed in the HERITAGE Family Study

	Name (unit)	Notes and sources
I: Steroids in the 19-carbon family (androstanes) and their derivatives		
Adrenal androgen precursors		
DHEA	Dehydroepiandrosterone (nmol/L)	Source: Adrenals
DELTA4	Androstenedione (nmol/L)	Source: Adrenals Intermediate in synthesis of TESTO, DHT, E2
DHEAS	DHEA sulfate (nmol/L)	Sulfated form of DHEA Most abundant steroid in circulation
DHEAE	DHEA fatty acid ester (nmol/L)	A second form of DHEA ester
Active androgens		
TESTO	Testosterone (nmol/L)	Source: Mainly by testicles
DHT	Dihydrotesterone (nmol/L)	Derived from TESTO or adrenal androgens precursors in multiple tissues
Androgen metabolites		
DIOLG	Androstane 3α17βdiol glucuronide (nmol/L)	Metabolite of TESTO and DHT
ADTG	Androsterone glucuronide (nmol/L)	Metabolite of TESTO and DHT
II: Pregnanes, Progestanes, and Estradiol		
PREGE	Pregnenolone fatty acid ester (nmol/L)	Derived from PREG in HDL particles and other sites
PROG	Progesterone (nmol/L)	Source: Mainly in the ovaries
OHPROG	17 hydroxy progesterone (nmol/L)	Derived from PROG in adrenals and gonads
E2	Estradiol (pmol/L)	Source: ovaries and other tissues
III: Aldosterone, Cortisol, SHBG and FAI		
ALDO	Aldosterone (nmol/L)	Source: adrenal cortex
CORT	Cortisol (nmol/L)	Source: adrenal cortex
SHBG	Sex hormone binding globulin (nmol/L)	Peptide transporting TESTO and E2 Source: mainly liver
FAI	Free androgen index	Calculated as TESTO/SHBG * 100

transformation of the hormones and their precursors. On 2 consecutive days, two blood samples were obtained after a 12-h fast pre- and post- exercise program. For eumenorrheic women, all samples were obtained in the early follicular phase of the menstrual cycle. None of the women of reproductive age had dramatically irregular menstrual cycles, as determined by questionnaire and during an interview. After centrifugation, aliquots were frozen at −80 °C. For nonconjugated steroids (see Table 1 for abbreviations), ALDO, dehydroepiandrosterone (DHEA) and testosterone (TESTO) were differentially extracted with hexane-ethyl acetate. Petroleum ether was used for the extraction of androstenedione (DELTA4) and dihydrotesterone (DHT). In-house RIAs were used to measure the levels of these four steroids. Progesterone, 17 hydroxy progesterone (OHPROG), cortisol (CORT), estradiol (E2), and DHEA sulfate (DHEAS) were assayed using commercial kits (Diagnostics Systems Lab, Webster, TX, USA). For glucuronide [androsterone glucuronide (ADTG) and androstane 3α17βdiol glucuronide (DIOLG)] and ester [DHEA fatty acid ester (DHEAE) and prenenolone fatty acid ester (PREGE)] conjugated steroids, ethanol extraction was performed, followed by C18 column chromatography. Glucuronide conjugates were submitted to hydrolysis with β-glucuronidase (Sigma Co., St. Louis, MO, USA). Fatty acid derivatives were submitted to saponification. Steroids were then separated by elution on LH-20 columns and measured by RIA. SHBG was determined with an IRMA-Count solid phase immunoradiometric assay using 125I (Diagnostics Systems Laboratories, Inc.). All assays were performed in the laboratory of Dr. Alain Belanger, Molecular Endocrinology, Laval University Medical Center (CHUL), Québec, Canada.

Statistical Analysis

The present study is based on sedentary adults from the HERITAGE Family Study who had complete baseline hormonal data. The mean of two measurements both before and after the exercise program has been used for all hormones and SHBG levels. Data of men and women were analyzed separately. Pearson product-moment correlation coefficients were used to quantify the relationships between baseline VO_2max (after adjustment for age and ethnicity) and its exercise training response (after adjustment for baseline, age and ethnicity) with fasting plasma steroid hormone, SHBG concentrations and the free androgen index (FAI). ANCOVA was used to compare each steroid, SHBG and FAI across quartiles of baseline VO_2max or its training response, with age and ethnicity as covariates. ANCOVA was used to compare the difference between the lowest 5% of the TESTO distribution and the men in the fourth quartile and between the highest 5% of the E2 distribution versus the women in the first quartile, with age and ethnicity as covariates. All analyses were performed using the SAS statistical package (SAS Institute, Inc., Cary, NC). Significance level was set at a more conservative p-value threshold of <0.01.

Table 2 Reproducibility of fasting steroid hormone levels in three HERITAGE ancillary studies

| | Intraclass correlation coefficient | | | | | |
| | Reliability of assay[a] | | HERITAGE test-retest[b] | | Three-day quality control[c] | |
	Males (N = 35)	Females (N = 25)	Males (N = 325)	Females (N = 420)	Males (N = 35)	Females (N = 25)
ADTG	0.81	0.95	0.91	0.93	0.77	0.96
ALDO	0.95	0.97	0.70	0.75	0.79	0.40
CORT	0.98	0.96	0.52	0.88	0.55	0.70
DELTA4	0.97	0.98	0.91	0.94	0.95	0.93
DHEA	0.97	0.97	0.76	0.80	0.86	0.71
DHEAE	0.77	0.94	0.79	0.85	0.79	0.82
DHEAS	0.97	0.98	0.96	0.97	0.94	0.92
DHT	0.96	0.86	0.93	0.83	0.95	0.86
DIOLG	0.80	0.97	0.96	0.93	0.73	0.98
E2	0.91	0.98	0.59	0.84	0.86	N/A
OHPROG	0.98	0.96	0.86	0.80	0.90	0.74
PREGE	0.89	0.87	0.83	0.86	0.69	0.79
PROG	0.92	0.99	0.90	0.84	0.79	N/A
SHBG	0.98	0.99	0.97	0.97	0.98	0.98
TESTO	0.97	0.95	0.95	0.90	0.95	0.92

[a]Repeated assays from the same aliquot. Samples from women obtained in the early follicular phase
[b]Test-retest from sample drawn on two different days. Samples from women obtained in the early follicular phase
[c]From samples tested three times in 3 weeks; menstrual cycle phase was not controlled in the female sample

Results

In the HERITAGE Family Study research program, three ancillary studies focusing on the within-subject variance and the reproducibility of test data were executed. Table 2 summarizes the main findings from these three sources for the steroid hormones and SHBG concentrations using the intraclass coefficients for repeated measures. In study 1, each assay was repeated from samples drawn from the same aliquot. Blood samples were drawn in the fasted state and those from eumenorrheic women were obtained in the early follicular phase. In study 2, the test-retest data were from samples drawn on two different days in the fasted state. Again, samples from eumenorrheic women were obtained in the early follicular phase. In study 3, samples were drawn in the fasted state three times in 3 weeks. However, the menstrual cycle phase was not controlled for in the female sample of the latter study. Globally, the results of these reproducibility studies indicate that the within-subject variation in hormone and SHBG levels was quite small compared to the between-subject fluctuations. The assays were quite reliable, as revealed by the very high intraclass coefficients for repeated assays on samples drawn from the same aliquot.

Table 3 Basic characteristics of sedentary males and females

	Men			Women		
	N	Age	BMI (kg/m²)	N	Age	BMI (kg/m²)
All	244	36 ± 14	26.5 ± 4.4	244	35 ± 14	25.1 ± 25.0
Blacks	61	33 ± 11	26.7 ± 4.1	59	33 ± 12	27.2 ± 5.8
Whites	183	37 ± 15	26.4 ± 4.5	185	35 ± 14	24.5 ± 4.6
17–29 years	114	23 ± 4	24.7 ± 4.3	121	22 ± 3	23.5 ± 4.8
30–49 years	74	40 ± 7	28.3 ± 3.7	75	41 ± 6	25.8 ± 4.4
50–65 years	56	56 ± 4	27.8 ± 4.3	48	55 ± 4	28.0 ± 5.0

Mean ± SD

This finding is particularly true for the steroids of high interest in the present paper, such as DHEA and DHEAS with coefficients >0.97, DHT and TESTO >0.86, E2 and PROG >0.91 and SHBG >0.95, all in both genders. When the day-to-day variation (plus the technical error of the assays) was considered in studies 2 and 3, all coefficients were high (>0.70), with the notable exception of CORT in males (~0.50).

Table 3 shows the physical characteristics of subjects stratified on the basis of age, gender and ethnicity. There were 244 adult subjects for each gender. About 25% of the subjects were blacks, with no difference between men and women. The male cohort was slightly overweight and heavier than the females, with the exception of black women.

Table 4 shows the baseline value of steroid hormones and SHBG in men and women. Mean and median values plus 95% confidence intervals and intervals between the first and fourth quartiles of the distributions are presented. Testing for skewness of distributions revealed that there was no indication of a major skewness problem with any of the variables.

Table 5 describes the VO_2max at baseline and training response. Shown are baseline VO_2max per kg of body weight and kg of fat-free mass. The most important inclusion criterion of the HERITAGE participants was that they needed to be confirmed sedentary. The low levels of CRF measured in males and females of this HERITAGE subsample confirm that they were indeed very sedentary as a group: with a mean age of about 35 years, VO_2max/kg weight reached only 36 ml O_2/kg in males and 28 in females.

Overall, steroid hormone levels were weakly associated with CRF in men but almost not at all in women. Table 6 summarizes the associations in men. Shown are partial correlations (controlling for age and ethnicity) between baseline plasma steroid hormone levels and baseline VO_2max/kg body weight, as well as hormonal levels (adjusted for age and ethnicity) by quartiles of fitness in men. There were substantial differences across the four quartiles of fitness, with Q1 having a mean VO_2max/kg weight value of 26.5 (SD = 2.3) and Q4 a mean of 48.4 (SD = 3.5). Significant partial correlations and significant differences across the four quartiles of VO_2max/kg were consistently found for ADTG, ALDO, DHT, OHPROG, SHBG, and TESTO. The patterns of differences across the fitness quartiles are depicted for DHT, OHPROG, TESTO and SHBG in Fig. 1, with indications of specific group comparison differences. Males with the lowest TESTO levels (lowest

Table 4 Steroid hormone levels at baseline in adult males and females

	Men (N = 244)				Women (N = 244)			
	Mean ± SD	95%CI	Median	Interquartile range	Mean ± SD	95%CI	Median	Interquartile range
ADTG	158 ± 87	−12–329	140	80	91 ± 54	−15–197	76	63
ALDO	0.3 ± 0.2	−0.0–0.6	0.2	0.2	0.3 ± 0.2	−0.1–0.6	0.2	0.2
CORT	376 ± 111	159–594	355	156	470 ± 241	−2–942	414	259
DELTA4	2.8 ± 1.5	0.1–5.6	2.7	1.8	2.4 ± 1.5	−0.5–5.3	2.1	2.1
DHEA	15.8 ± 10.3	−4.4–20.1	13.9	11.4	14.3 ± 10.2	−5.7–34.4	11.8	12.0
DHEAE	9.4 ± 5.8	−1.8–20.5	7.7	6.7	7.9 ± 5.4	−2.8–18.5	6.5	5.3
DHEAS	5696 ± 3172	−521–11913	5128	4538	3730 ± 2277	−734–8193	3202	2610
DHT	2.8 ± 1.2	0.3–5.2	2.7	1.8	0.5 ± 0.3	0.0–1.0	0.5	0.4
DIOLG	28.7 ± 14.0	1.3–56.0	26.7	13.1	14.1 ± 7.7	1.1–29.2	12.2	8.3
E2	72 ± 45	−17–161	66	47	136 ± 195	−246–518	82	108.2
OHPRG	5.5 ± 2.9	−0.2–11.1	5.1	3.5	2.1 ± 1.4	−0.7–4.8	1.8	1.4
PREGE	16.8 ± 9.6	−2.1–35.6	14.0	12.1	13.9 ± 9.1	−3.9–31.7	10.9	11.0
PROG	1.7 ± 0.8	0.–3.3	1.6	0.7	1.6 ± 3.0	−4.3–7.5	1.2	1.2
SHBG	39.5 ± 16.6	7.2–71.7	36.9	25.0	86.4 ± 49.8	−11.2–184.0	70.7	53.3
TESTO	15.1 ± 6.1	3.–27.0	14.8	9.0	1.3 ± 0.7	0.0–2.6	1.2	0.7
FAI	43.1 ± 21.3	1.4–84.8	39.1	25.3	2.0 ± 1.4	−0.7–4.7	1.6	1.6

Units of steroid hormone and SHBG were nmol/L except E2 (pmol/L). Unit of FAI is in %

Table 5 VO_2max at baseline and its training response in adult males and females of HERITAGE study

	Men (N = 244)				Women (N = 244)			
	X ± SD	95%CI	Median	Interquartile range	X ± SD	95%CI	Median	Interquartile range
VO_2max (ml/min/kg BW)	36.3 ± 8.6	19.4–53.2	35.3	13.4	28.3 ± 6.9	14.8–41.8	28.7	10.3
VO_2max (ml/min/kg FFM)	46.5 ± 7.3	32.2–60.8	46.1	10.6	40.7 ± 6.4	28.2–53.2	41.3	9.2
$\triangle VO_2$max (ml/min)[a]	453 ± 234	−5–911	448	321	347 ± 177	−1–694	338	233

BW body weight, *FFM* fat-free mass

[a]Unadjusted data

Table 6 Partial correlations between baseline plasma steroid hormone levels, baseline VO_2max/kg body weight, and hormonal levels by quartiles of fitness in men

	Partial correlation coefficients[a]	Quartiles[b]				F, P for trend[c]
		Q1	Q2	Q3	Q4	
VO_2max/kg BW		26.5 ± 2.3	32.0 ± 1.7	38.5 ± 2.4	48.4 ± 3.5	
Ages		49 ± 11	41 ± 13	31 ± 11	23 ± 6	
Ethnicity		67% (white)	75% (white)	64% (white)	93% (white)	
ADTG	−0.18*	181.1 ± 12.3	172.7 ± 10.5	155.0 ± 10.5	123.4 ± 12.7	3.11, p = 0.0272
ALDO	0.19*	0.24 ± 0.02	0.25 ± 0.02	0.24 ± 0.02	0.33 ± 0.02	**3.83, P = 0.0105**
CORT	0.14	355 ± 16	361 ± 14	383 ± 14	407 ± 17	1.40, p = 0.2435
DELT4	0.12	2.5 ± 0.2	2.7 ± 0.2	2.8 ± 0.2	3.1 ± 0.2	1.25, p = 0.2906
DHEA	0.00	15.2 ± 1.4	15.1 ± 1.2	16.9 ± 1.2	15.9 ± 1.4	0.42, p = 0.7386
DHEAE	−0.12	10.2 ± 0.8	9.5 ± 0.7	9.2 ± 0.7	8.5 ± 0.9	0.51, p = 0.6725
DHEAS	−0.01	5299 ± 424	5877 ± 359	5655 ± 359	5551 ± 437	0.48, p = 0.6951
DHT	0.26***	2.2 ± 0.2	2.6 ± 0.1	3.0 ± 0.1	3.2 ± 0.2	**14.93, P < 0.0001**
DIOLG	−0.12	30.3 ± 2.1	29.6 ± 1.8	29.9 ± 1.8	24.9 ± 2.1	1.32, p = 0.2677
E2	0.03	72.7 ± 7.0	66.3 ± 5.9	73.1 ± 5.9	76.5 ± 7.2	0.82, p = 0.4817
OHPROG	0.25***	4.5 ± 0.4	4.8 ± 0.3	6.1 ± 0.3	6.5 ± 0.4	**15.47, P < 0.0001**
PREGE	−0.01	15.9 ± 1.4	17.1 ± 1.2	18.4 ± 1.2	15.6 ± 1.5	1.15, p = 0.3299
PROG	0.11	1.4 ± 0.1	1.7 ± 0.1	1.8 ± 0.1	1.8 ± 0.1	2.37, p = 0.0713
SHBG	0.30***	32.6 ± 2.4	37.0 ± 2.0	39.3 ± 2.0	49.1 ± 2.4	**6.46, p = 0.0003**
TESTO	0.34***	11.5 ± 0.9	13.4 ± 0.7	16.9 ± 0.7	18.6 ± 0.9	**9.94, P < 0.0001**
FAI	−0.08	43.3 ± 2.9	41.6 ± 2.5	48.3 ± 2.5	39.2 ± 3.0	2.45, p = 0.0645

Units of steroid hormone and SHBG are nmol/L except E2 (pmol/L). Unit of FAI is in %

The bold results have the highest significance levels

*P < 0.01; ***P < 0.0001

[a] Age and ethnicity were controlled for in the partial correlations between baseline plasma steroid hormone levels and baseline VO_2max/kg body weight

[b] Adjusted data for steroid hormone, SHBG, and FAI, mean ± SEM

[c] Age and ethnicity as covariates when comparing hormonal levels by quartiles of fitness in men; F = F ratio, P = p-value

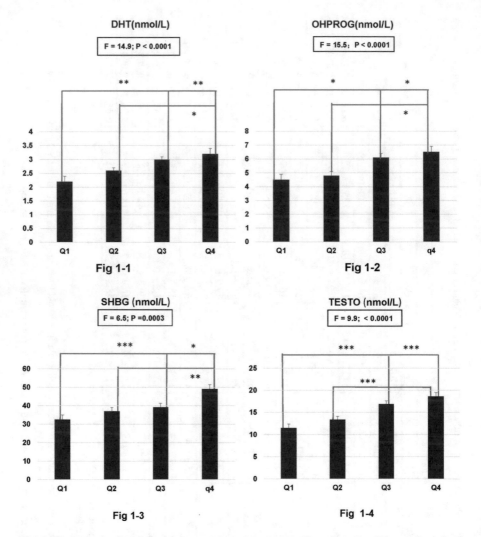

Fig. 1 Hormone levels adjusted for age and ethnicity by quartiles of baseline VO₂max/kg weight in men. Mean and SEM are shown. Dihydrotesterone (DHT), 17 hydroxy progesterone (OHPROG), sex hormone binding globulin (SHBG), testosterone (TESTO) *P < 0.01; **P < 0.001; ***P < 0.0001

5% of the distribution; N = 13; TESTO concentration <6.16 nmol/L) were compared to the subjects in the upper quartile of the TESTO distribution (N = 61; TESTO concentration >19.56 nmol/L) for potential differences in VO₂max. Significant gaps in CRF were observed, with the low TESTO subjects exhibiting lower VO₂max/kg BW (33.7 ± 1.4 vs. 39.9 ± 0.6, F = 15.2, P = 0.0002) and VO₂max/kg FFM (43.9 ± 1.3 vs. 48.3 ± 0.6, F = 9.3, P = 0.0032).

The same analyses were performed in the female sample and the results are shown in Table 7. Only FAI was significantly correlated (partial correlation) with

Table 7 Partial correlations between baseline plasma steroid hormone levels, baseline VO_2max/kg body weight and hormonal levels by quartiles of fitness in women

	Partial correlation coefficients[a]	Quartiles[b]				F, P for trend[c]
		Q1	Q2	Q3	Q4	
VO_2max/kg BW		19.7 ± 2.2	25.4 ± 2.0	30.7 ± 1.3	37.4 ± 2.8	
Ages		47 ± 11	38 ± 13	30 ± 10	23 ± 6	
Ethnicity		61% (white)	62% (white)	85% (white)	95% (white)	
ADTG	−0.08	98.3 ± 8.1	90.2 ± 6.9	91.6 ± 6.9	83.7 ± 8.1	0.48, p = 0.6992
ALDO	0.15	0.23 ± 0.03	0.1 ± 0.02	0.22 ± 0.02	0.32 ± 0.03	3.68, p = 0.0128
CORT	0.14	409.3 ± 35	442 ± 29	525 ± 29	505 ± 34	1.95, p = 0.1215
DELT4	0.05	2.2 ± 0.2	2.5 ± 0.2	2.3 ± 0.2	2.5 ± 0.2	0.48, p = 0.6975
DHEA	0.01	14.9 ± 1.4	14.6 ± 1.2	13.3 ± 1.2	14.6 ± 1.4	0.36, p = 0.7841
DHEAE	−0.06	9.3 ± 0.8	8.5 ± 0.7	6.2 ± 0.7	7.5 ± 0.8	2.72, p = 0.0452
DHEAS	−0.04	3954 ± 314	3843 ± 265	3455 ± 265	3667 ± 312	0.49, P = 0.6919
DHT	−0.04	0.54 ± 0.04	0.59 ± 0.03	0.48 ± 0.03	0.48 ± 0.04	2.19, p = 0.0897
DIOLG	−0.08	15.1 ± 1.2	14.9 ± 1.0	13.6 ± 1.0	12.6 ± 1.2	1.25, p = 0.2922
E2	−0.04	155 ± 31	132 ± 26	150 ± 26	107 ± 30	2.46, p = 0.0636
OHPROG	0.02	2.4 ± 0.2	1.8 ± 0.2	1.8 ± 0.2	2.1 ± 0.2	2.06, p = 0.1064
PREGE	−0.05	16.1 ± 1.4	14.1 ± 1.2	12.1 ± 1.2	13.4 ± 1.4	1.43, p = 0.2353
PROG	−0.02	2.2 ± 0.5	1.5 ± 0.4	1.2 ± 0.4	1.4 ± 0.5	0.79, p = 0.5002
SHBG	0.14	66.7 ± 7.8	86.0 ± 6.6	101.3 ± 6.6	91.7 ± 7.7	3.41, p = 0.0183
TESTO	−0.04	1.3 ± 0.1	1.4 ± 0.1	1.3 ± 0.1	1.2 ± 0.1	1.01, p = 0.3889
FAI	−0.20*	2.6 ± 0.2	2.2 ± 0.2	1.5 ± 0.2	1.5 ± 0.2	**4.45, p = 0.0046**

Units of steroid hormone and SHBG are nmol/L except E2 (pmol/L). Unit of FAI is in %
*$P < 0.01$
[a]Age and ethnicity as adjustment factors for partial correlation between baseline plasma steroid hormone levels and baseline VO_2max/kg body weight
[b]Adjusted data for steroid hormone, SHBG, and FAI, mean ± SEM
[c]Age and ethnicity as covariance when comparing hormonal levels by quartiles of fitness in women; F = F ratio, P = p-value

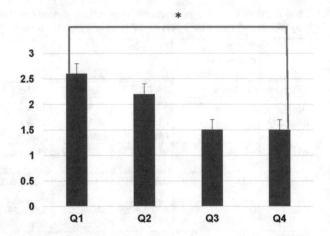

Fig. 2 Free androgen index (FAI) adjusted for age and ethnicity by quartiles of baseline VO$_2$max/kg weight in women. Mean and SEM are shown. $\underline{F = 4.5}$; *P = 0.05

baseline VO$_2$max/kg weight and differed across the four fitness groups. None of the hormones was consistently associated with fitness in women. The FAI values across the four fitness quartiles are depicted in Fig. 2.

Baseline plasma steroid levels, SHBG concentrations and FAI were not associated with the gains in VO$_2$max resulting from exposure to the 20-week aerobic exercise program in men or in women. For the latter analyses, the gains in VO$_2$max in mlO$_2$ were adjusted for baseline level, age and ethnicity. Notably, the men in the low TESTO group (lowest 5% of the distribution) did not show a deficit in CRF responsiveness to exercise training (results not shown).

Discussion

The present study is the most comprehensive report published to date on the relationships between a large panel of plasma steroid hormones and CRF in sedentary men and women at baseline and in response to a fully standardized and monitored 20-week exercise program. Of particular significance, the plasma concentrations of steroid hormones were measured twice in the morning in a fasted state (samples from two different days) before and again twice (from samples obtained on 2 days) after the exercise training program. Also of significance, all blood samples were drawn in the early follicular phase of the menstrual cycle for eumenorrheic women. Furthermore, three quality-control studies were implemented to quantify the magnitude of the assay variance and the within-individual day-to-day variation in hormone concentrations. As a large number of tests of significance were performed, an alpha threshold of $p < 0.01$ was used to reduce the risk of false positive results.

Significant associations were found by partial correlation analyses between baseline VO$_2$max/kg weight and plasma levels of ADTG, ALDO, DHT, OHPROG, SHBG, and TESTO in men. In contrast, in women, only the FAI was significantly associated with baseline VO$_2$max/kg weight. When comparing steroids, SHBG and

FAI across quartiles of baseline VO_2max ml/kg weight, the plasma concentration of DHT, OHPROG, SHBG, and TESTO increased gradually from Q1 to Q4 in men whereas FAI progressively decreased as fitness increased in women, indicating that a higher level of TESTO was associated with better CRF. Indeed, once the effects of age and ethnicity were taken into account, TESTO explained about 3% of the variance in baseline VO_2max/kg weight in men. In females, FAI also accounted for about 3% of the baseline VO_2max/kg weight, with the same statistical control over age and ethnicity. Baseline plasma steroid levels, SHBG concentrations or FAI were not associated with the gains in VO_2max resulting from exposure to the 20-week aerobic exercise program after adjustment for baseline values, age and ethnicity.

The present results reinforce the idea that SHBG[3] and TESTO (Storer et al. 2016) are weakly correlated with baseline fitness. In the CARDIA Male Hormone Study (391 blacks and 604 whites, aged 24–32 years), SHBG was significantly (p = 0.05) associated with estimated CRF among white men, with quartiles four and two having the highest (33.5 nmol/L) and lowest (27.8 nmol/L) SHBG concentrations, respectively (Wolin et al. 2007). TESTO supplementation in mobility-limited older men (n = 64) increased hemoglobin and attenuated the age-related declines in VO_2peak (Storer et al. 2016). However, our results also contradict those of other reports. Lucertini et al. (2015) found basal CORT levels were lower in the high-fit (VO_2max, 37.9 ± 0.9 ml/kg/min) than the low-fit group (VO_2max, 26.4 ± 0.7 ml/kg/min). We could not herein confirm the relationship between CORT and fitness. This discrepancy may be explained by the basic characteristics of the study designs: for instance, VO_2max was estimated using the Rockport Walking Test in the study of Lucertini et al. (2015), the sample size of their study was quite small and subjects were older (*n* = 22, mean age 68 years), and CORT was assayed from saliva samples obtained at 18:00, late afternoon. Huang et al. also did not find a difference in CORT between high-fitness (VO_2max, 51.0 ± 0.8, ml/kg/min, ages: 22.3 ± 1.97, n = 7) and low-fitness groups (VO_2max, 36.3 ± 1.3, ml/kg/min, ages, 20.9 ± 0.8, n = 7) in males (Huang et al. 2014).

The World Anti-Doping Agency (WADA) has developed a specific steroid module as a part of their Athlete Biological Passport (ABP; Alladio et al. 2016), which was implemented internationally in January 2014. Anabolic steroids represent the most abundant class of substance used to enhance performance in elite sports. Anabolic steroids are generally used to enhance muscle mass and muscular strength or power. Their use for improvement of endurance performance or recovery from training is less frequent. Our three quality control studies of plasma levels of steroids revealed that their blood concentrations were quite stable within an individual. We observed that TESTO and DHT were weakly but positively associated with CRF in men only. These associations were lost when VO_2max was adjusted for fat-free mass (results not shown here), suggesting that the associations with fitness may have been mediated by the muscle mass and not by the ability to deliver oxygen (cardiac output and hemoglobin content of blood) to the working muscle. Importantly, there was no relation between plasma levels of steroids and the VO_2max training response to the HERITAGE exercise program. Globally, our results provide little support for a substantial role of high plasma steroids content in CRF and endurance performance.

We conclude from our detailed observations that baseline plasma steroid levels are only weakly associated with individual differences in CRF in the sedentary state in men, whereas no association could be detected with trainability, as defined by the change in VO_2max with the exercise program. The associations are particularly consistent for the plasma concentrations of testosterone and SHBG. In women, the most consistent association pattern was seen with the FAI, potentially reflecting the fact that high levels of free testosterone in females could be associated with slightly elevated CRF.

Acknowledgments The HERITAGE Family Study has been supported over the years by multiple grants from the National Institute for Heart, Lung and Blood Diseases of the National Institutes of Health (HL45670, C. Bouchard and T. Rankinen; HL47323, A.S. Leon; HL47317, D.C. Rao; HL47327, J.S. Skinner; HL47321, J.H. Wilmore, deceased). CB is partially funded by the John W. Barton Sr. Chair in Genetics and Nutrition. Zihong HE is funded by the China Scholarship Council (File No. 201603620001) and China Institute of Sport Science (2015-01, 2016-01). We would like to express our gratitude to Dr. Alain Belanger (retired) and his staff from the Molecular Endocrinology Laboratory of the Laval University Medical Center in Quebec City, Canada, for the assays of the steroids and their dedication to the HERITAGE Family Study.

Disclosures AT receives research funding from Johnson & Johnson Medical Companies for studies unrelated to the present paper.

References

Alladio E, Caruso R, Gerace E, Amante E, Salomone A, Vincenti M (2016) Application of multivariate statistics to the steroidal module of the athlete biological passport: a proof of concept study. Anal Chim Acta 922:19–29

Bouchard C, Leon AS, Rao DC, Skinner JS, Wilmore JH, Gagnon J (1995) The HERITAGE family study. Aims, design, and measurement protocol. Med Sci Sports Exerc 27:721–729

Bouchard C, Blair SN, Katzmarzyk PT (2015) Less sitting, more physical activity, or higher fitness? Mayo Clin Proc 90:1533–1540

Bruder-Nascimento T, Ferreira NS, Zanotto CZ, Ramalho F, Pequeno IO, Olivon VC, Neves KB, Alves-Lopes R, Campos E, Silva CA, Fazan R, Carlos D, Mestriner FL, Prado D, Pereira FV, Braga T, Luiz JP, Cau SB, Elias PC, Moreira AC, Camara NO, Zamboni DS, Alves-Filho JC, Tostes RC (2016) NLRP3 inflammasome mediates aldosterone-induced vascular damage. Circulation 134:1866–1880

Canoy D, Barber TM, Pouta A, Hartikainen AL, McCarthy MI, Franks S, Jarvelin MR, Tapanainen JS, Ruokonen A, Huhtaniemi IT, Martikainen H (2014) Serum sex hormone-binding globulin and testosterone in relation to cardiovascular disease risk factors in young men: a population-based study. Eur J Endocrinol 170:863–872

Couillard C, Gagnon J, Bergeron J, Leon AS, Rao DC, Skinner JS, Wilmore JH, Despres JP, Bouchard C (2000) Contribution of body fatness and adipose tissue distribution to the age variation in plasma steroid hormone concentrations in men: the HERITAGE family study. J Clin Endocrinol Metab 85:1026–1031

Engberg E, Alen M, Kukkonen-Harjula K, Peltonen JE, Tikkanen HO, Pekkarinen H (2012) Life events and change in leisure time physical activity: a systematic review. Sports Med 42:433–447

Ennour-Idrissi K, Maunsell E, Diorio C (2015) Effect of physical activity on sex hormones in women: a systematic review and meta-analysis of randomized controlled trials. Breast Cancer Res 17:139

Group ECW (2006) Hormones and cardiovascular health in women. Hum Reprod Update 12:483–497

Haddock BL, Marshak HP, Mason JJ, Blix G (2000) The effect of hormone replacement therapy and exercise on cardiovascular disease risk factors in postmenopausal women. Sports Med 29:39–49

Hammond GL (2016) Plasma steroid-binding proteins: primary gatekeepers of steroid hormone action. J Endocrinol 230:R13–R25

Hasan KM, Rahman MS, Arif KM, Sobhani ME (2012) Psychological stress and aging: role of glucocorticoids (GCs). Age 34:1421–1433

Huang CJ, Webb HE, Beasley KN, McAlpine DA, Tangsilsat SE, Acevedo EO (2014) Cardiorespiratory fitness does not alter plasma pentraxin 3 and cortisol reactivity to acute psychological stress and exercise. Appl Physiol Nutr Metab 39:375–380

Kim JW, Kim DY (2012) Effects of aerobic exercise training on serum sex hormone binding globulin, body fat index, and metabolic syndrome factors in obese postmenopausal women. Metab Syndr Relat Disord 10:452–457

Kohl HW 3rd, Craig CL, Lambert EV, Inoue S, Alkandari JR, Leetongin G, Kahlmeier S, Lancet Physical Activity Series Working G (2012) The pandemic of physical inactivity: global action for public health. Lancet 380:294–305

Kumagai H, Zempo-Miyaki A, Yoshikawa T, Tsujimoto T, Tanaka K, Maeda S (2016) Increased physical activity has a greater effect than reduced energy intake on lifestyle modification-induced increases in testosterone. J Clin Biochem Nutr 58:84–89

Labrie F (2015) All sex steroids are made intracellularly in peripheral tissues by the mechanisms of intracrinology after menopause. J Steroid Biochem Mol Biol 145:133–138

Lee IM, Shiroma EJ, Lobelo F, Puska P, Blair SN, Katzmarzyk PT, Lancet Physical Activity Series Working G (2012) Effect of physical inactivity on major non-communicable diseases worldwide: an analysis of burden of disease and life expectancy. Lancet 380:219–229

Lother A, Moser M, Bode C, Feldman RD, Hein L (2015) Mineralocorticoids in the heart and vasculature: new insights for old hormones. Annu Rev Pharmacol Toxicol 55:289–312

Lucertini F, Ponzio E, Di Palma M, Galati C, Federici A, Barbadoro P, D'Errico MM, Prospero E, Ambrogini P, Cuppini R, Lattanzi D, Minelli A (2015) High cardiorespiratory fitness is negatively associated with daily cortisol output in healthy aging men. PLoS One 10:e0141970

Luu-The V, Labrie F (2010) The intracrine sex steroid biosynthesis pathways. Prog Brain Res 181:177–192

Meyer MR, Barton M (2016) Estrogens and coronary artery disease: new clinical perspectives. Adv Pharmacol 77:307–360

Meyer EJ, Nenke MA, Rankin W, Lewis JG, Torpy DJ (2016) Corticosteroid-binding globulin: a review of basic and clinical advances. Hormon-Stoffwechselforsch 48:359–371

Nicolaides NC, Kyratzi E, Lamprokostopoulou A, Chrousos GP, Charmandari E (2015) Stress, the stress system and the role of glucocorticoids. Neuroimmunomodulation 22:6–19

Pongkan W, Chattipakorn SC, Chattipakorn N (2016) Roles of testosterone replacement in cardiac ischemia-reperfusion injury. J Cardiovasc Pharmacol Ther 21:27–43

Reslan OM, Khalil RA (2012) Vascular effects of estrogenic menopausal hormone therapy. Rev Recent Clin Trials 7:47–70

Sarzynski MA, Ghosh S, Bouchard C (2016) Genomic and transcriptomic predictors of response levels to endurance exercise training. J Physiol. https://doi.org/10.1113/JP272559

Sato K, Lemitsu M (2015) Exercise and sex steroid hormones in skeletal muscle. J Steroid Biochem Mol Biol 145:200–205

Sato K, Lemitsu M, Matsutani K, Kurihara T, Hamaoka T, Fujita S (2014) Resistance training restores muscle sex steroid hormone steroidogenesis in older men. FASEB J 28:1891–1897

Singh R, Artaza JN, Taylor WE, Braga M, Yuan X, Gonzalez-Cadavid NF, Bhasin S (2006) Testosterone inhibits adipogenic differentiation in 3T3-L1 cells: nuclear translocation of androgen receptor complex with beta-catenin and T-cell factor 4 may bypass canonical Wnt signaling to down-regulate adipogenic transcription factors. Endocrinology 147:141–154

Sinha-Hikim I, Taylor WE, Gonzalez-Cadavid NF, Zheng W, Bhasin S (2004) Androgen receptor in human skeletal muscle and cultured muscle satellite cells: up-regulation by androgen treatment. J Clin Endocrinol Metab 89:5245–5255

Siri WE (1956) The gross composition of the body. Adv Biol Med Phys 4:239–280

Skinner JS, Wilmore KM, Krasnoff JB, Jaskolski A, Jaskolska A, Gagnon J, Province MA, Leon AS, Rao DC, Wilmore JH, Bouchard C (2000) Adaptation to a standardized training program and changes in fitness in a large, heterogeneous population: the HERITAGE Family Study. Med Sci Sports Exerc 32:157–161

Skinner JS, Jaskolski A, Jaskolska A, Krasnoff J, Gagnon J, Leon AS, Rao DC, Wilmore JH, Bouchard C, Study HF (2001) Age, sex, race, initial fitness, and response to training: the HERITAGE Family Study. J Appl Physiol 90:1770–1776

Storer TW, Bhasin S, Travison TG, Pencina K, Miciek R, McKinnon J, Basaria S (2016) Testosterone attenuates age-related fall in aerobic function in mobility limited older men with low testosterone. J Clin Endocrinol Metab 101:2562–2569

Ukkola O, Gagnon J, Rankinen T, Thompson PA, Hong Y, Leon AS, Rao DC, Skinner JS, Wilmore JH, Bouchard C (2001) Age, body mass index, race and other determinants of steroid hormone variability: the HERITAGE Family Study. Eur J Endocrinol 145:1–9

United States Department of Health and Human Services (2008) 2008 physical activity guidelines for Americans: be active, healthy, and happy! U.S. Dept. of Health and Human Services, Washington, DC

Wilmore JH, Stanforth PR, Domenick MA, Gagnon J, Daw EW, Leon AS, Rao DC, Skinner JS, Bouchard C (1997) Reproducibility of anthropometric and body composition measurements: the HERITAGE Family Study. Intl J Obes Rel Metab Disord 21:297–303

Wolin KY, Colangelo LA, Liu K, Sternfeld B, Gapstur SM (2007) Associations of androgens with physical activity and fitness in young black and white men: the CARDIA Male Hormone Study. Prev Med 44:426–431

Sending the Signal: Muscle Glycogen Availability as a Regulator of Training Adaptation

Check for updates

John A. Hawley

Abstract Exercise training-induced adaptations in human skeletal muscle are largely determined by the mode, volume, intensity and frequency of the training stimulus. However, a growing body of evidence demonstrates that the availability of endogenous and exogenous macronutrients can modify multiple intramuscular responses to both endurance- and resistance-based exercise. Acutely manipulating substrate availability (by altering diet composition and/or timing of meals) rapidly alters the concentration of blood-borne substrates and hormones that modulate several receptor-mediated signaling pathways. The release of cytokines and growth factors from contracting skeletal muscle also stimulates cell surface receptors and activates many intracellular signaling cascades. These local and systemic factors cause marked perturbations in the storage profile of skeletal muscle (and other insulin-sensitive tissues) that, in turn, exert pronounced effects on resting fuel metabolism and patterns of fuel utilization during exercise. When repeated over weeks and months, such nutrient-exercise interactions have the potential to alter numerous adaptive processes in skeletal muscle that ultimately drive the phenotype-specific variability observed between individuals. One strategy that augments endurance-training adaptation is commencing exercise with low muscle glycogen concentration ("train-low"). The amplified training response observed with low endogenous carbohydrate availability is likely regulated by enhanced activation of key cell signalling kinases (e.g., AMPK, p38MAPK), transcription factors (e.g., p53, PPARδ) and transcriptional co-activators (e.g., PGC-1α), such that a coordinated up-regulation of both the nuclear and mitochondrial genomes occurs. This chapter provides a contemporary perspective of our understanding of the molecular and cellular events that take place in skeletal muscle in response to exercise commenced after alterations in nutrient availability and discusses how the ensuing hor-

J. A. Hawley (✉)
Mary MacKillop Institute for Health Research, Australian Catholic University, Melbourne, VIC, Australia

Research Institute for Sport and Exercise Sciences, Liverpool John Moores University, Liverpool, UK
e-mail: john.hawley@acu.edu.au

43

monal milieu interacts with specific contractile stimulus to modulate many of the acute responses to exercise, thereby potentially promoting or inhibiting subsequent training adaptation.

Introduction

Classic studies conducted in the late nineteenth and early twentieth century determined that the fuels that supported contracting skeletal muscle during continuous exercise lasting longer than several minutes were intra- and extra-muscular carbohydrate and lipid substrates, with only a minor contribution from amino acids (for review, see Hawley et al. 2015). During this time, it was also demonstrated that manipulation of the macronutrient content of the preceding diet resulted in marked changes in the time for which exercise at a fixed, submaximal power output could be sustained; furthermore, subjects perceived exercise to be easier after several days of a high carbohydrate diet than when the preceding diet was low in carbohydrate and high in fat (Hawley et al. 2015). In the mid twentieth century, a large body of work, mainly undertaken in laboratories in Europe, extended the earlier observations of the importance of carbohydrate-based fuels for prolonged, intense exercise.

The period from 1960 up until the late 1980s has been termed the "classical period" of exercise biochemistry (Brooks and Mercier 1994). With remarkable foresight, Goldstein (1961) proposed that a "humoral factor" was liberated by muscle during contraction that "activates the glucose transport system" and helps "regulate carbohydrate metabolism" in what was later to become known as "muscle cross talk." At the beginning of the 1960s, little was known about the regulation of mitochondrial biogenesis in skeletal muscle in response to exercise training. However, seminal work by Holloszy (1967) heralded a major advance in unravelling some of the cellular events controlling muscle bioenergetics in response to exercise. It was during this time that the percutaneous needle biopsy technique was introduced into exercise biochemistry (Bergström and Hultman 1966), making it possible to conduct invasive studies and determine the impact of training, diet, and other manipulations on selected metabolic characteristics. Studies conducted in labs in Europe and North America advanced our understanding of the impact of training and diet manipulations on muscle substrate stores, the interactive effects of exercise and orally administered carbohydrate on muscle glucose kinetics and exercise capacity, and the protein synthetic response to exercise (Hawley et al. 2015; Brooks and Mercier 1994). New insights into the influence of substrate availability on the hormonal response to prolonged exercise were also advanced in this period (Galbo et al. 1979). At the same time, major progress in our knowledge of how exercise activates cellular, molecular, and biochemical pathways with regulatory roles in training response adaptation took place, and skeletal muscle was confirmed to have endocrine-like effects, releasing cytokines and other peptides to orchestrate inter-organ "cross talk" (Pedersen et al. 2003).

During the past two decades, exercise training-induced adaptations in skeletal muscle have been shown to be the result of the cumulative effects of the acute responses to repeated, single exercise bouts (Perry et al. 2010), with the rapid and transient changes in gene transcription following a single bout of exercise leading to chronic effects on protein expression when repeated over time. However, only recently have we begun to appreciate the impact that alterations in substrate availability have on modifying training responses-adaptations. While substrates like carbohydrate and fat were viewed merely as energy stores for contracting muscles, we are now beginning to understand that fuel availability per se is a crucial regulator of many biochemical and cellular signaling events with roles in mitochondrial biogenesis, autophagy, health and performance. This chapter will provide a contemporary perspective of our understanding of the regulation of substrate metabolism; the molecular and cellular events that take place in skeletal muscle in response to exercise commenced after alterations in nutrient availability; and how the ensuing hormonal milieu interacts with specific contractile stimulus to modulate many of the acute responses to exercise, thereby potentially promoting or inhibiting subsequent training adaptation.

Fuels for the Fire: Patterns of Skeletal Muscle Fuel Utilization

Both carbohydrate- (muscle and liver glycogen, blood glucose, muscle and liver lactate) and fat- (adipose and intramuscular triglycerides, blood-borne free fatty acids and triglycerides) based fuels are important substrates for oxidative phosphorylation and energy production in skeletal muscle (Brooks and Mercier 1994). Compared to the finite stores of carbohydrate, endogenous lipid stores in humans are plentiful and represent a potentially unlimited source of fuel for skeletal muscle metabolism during aerobic exercise. However, fatty acid (FA) oxidation by muscle is limited, at least during the power outputs sustained by athletes during training and competition (Hawley and Leckey 2015). Unlike the oxidation of carbohydrate, which is closely geared to the energy requirements of the working muscle, there are no mechanisms for matching the availability and utilization of FA to the rate of energy expenditure (Holloszy et al. 1988). However, the oxidation of any one fuel or another at rest or during exercise does not occur in isolation and is typically the result of the integration of many metabolic signals involving exogenous and endogenous substrate availability, the prevailing hormonal milieu as well as muscle and whole-body energetic demands.

Both carbohydrate- and fat-based fuels are oxidized at rest to provide the energy required for basal metabolic processes in skeletal muscle, with a reciprocal relationship between the utilization of carbohydrate and fat: fuel shifts occurring at rest are largely driven by the availability of substrates and the concomitant hormonal environment (i.e., plasma glucose, insulin, FFA and glucagon concentrations) in the face of a generally unchanged metabolic demand. For example, increasing blood glucose availability by feeding of a carbohydrate-rich meal increases the uptake and oxidation of glucose into skeletal muscle while concomitantly decreasing the oxidation of fat; but overall, there is little change in resting metabolic rate. The decreased rate of FA oxidation at rest is largely attributable to a carbohydrate feeding-induced rise in insulin concentration that impairs lipolysis (i.e., the rate of appearance [Ra] of FFA into the systemic circulation), an effect that can persist for up to four hours after a carbohydrate-rich meal (Bonadonna et al. 1990).

The concept of a reciprocal relationship between fat and carbohydrate oxidation, at least in resting muscle, stemmed from the work of Randle and colleagues in the 1960s (Randle et al. 1964). Their experiments demonstrated that increased lipid availability [i.e., circulating plasma free fatty acids (FFA)] increased FA oxidation and decreased carbohydrate oxidation in muscle and that it was the increase in fat availability that resulted in key intracellular perturbations, including increased contents of muscle acetyl-coenzyme A (CoA), citrate, and glucose-6-phosphate: lipid-induced changes at these key regulatory sites decreased muscle carbohydrate metabolism. The results of these early studies, which subsequently formed the bases of the "glucose-fatty acid cycle" hypothesis (Randle 1986), were obtained by comparing supra-physiological levels of FFA while glucose concentration was "clamped." The prevailing paradigm was that carbohydrate-based substrates were the muscle's "default" fuel but that increased FA availability could "switch" muscle fuel use and down-regulate carbohydrate metabolism. While the "glucose-fatty acid cycle" proposed by Randle and coworkers (Randle et al. 1964) explained the mechanisms responsible for the down regulation of carbohydrate metabolism in the face of high FA availability, these researchers failed to perform the control or "crossover" experiments, in which FA availability was held constant but glucose levels were increased. This, apparently, was because they steadfastly believed that there was little regulation of fat metabolism in skeletal muscle at rest (or presumably during exercise) and that the key determinant of the rate of FA oxidation was simply a function of the availability of fat and its regulation at the level of the mitochondrial membranes through the carnitine-palmitoyl transferase (CPT) complex (Randle et al. 1964).

While there are situations in which the glucose-fatty acid cycle operates, a series of elegant studies conducted in the late 1990s clearly demonstrated that carbohydrate availability directly regulates fat oxidation at rest and during exercise (Coyle et al. 1997; Horowitz et al. 1997; Romijn et al. 1995). Coyle et al. (1997) demonstrated that a carbohydrate-rich meal that induced hyperglycemia and hyperinsulinemia increased glycolytic flux and directly reduced rates of FA oxidation during low-intensity exercise. Carbohydrate feeding reduced the Ra of plasma FFA by ~35%, resulting in a reduction in both plasma FFA and intramuscular triglyceride oxidation, suggesting a coordinated effect of increased glucose availability on adipose tissue and muscle. These observations indicate that glucose can directly regulate fat oxidation during exercise and that the classic "glucose-fatty acid cycle" proposed by Randle and colleagues (Randle 1986; Randle et al. 1964), in which fat availability alone regulates rates of FA oxidation, is an overly simplistic view of fuel regulation.

The concept that altering substrate availability can modify the proportions of carbohydrate and fat utilized by working muscle is certainly not new (Hawley et al. 2015). However, during the past decade, data from several independent laboratories has provided evidence that commencing selected exercise sessions under conditions of reduced carbohydrate availability can promote training-induced adaptations in human skeletal muscle to a greater magnitude than if the same sessions were commenced with normal or high glycogen levels.

Sending the Signal: The Training Response-Adaptation

The goals of endurance exercise training are to induce an array of physiological and metabolic adaptations that enable an individual to increase the rate of energy production from both aerobic and oxygen-independent pathways, maintain tighter metabolic control (i.e., match ATP production with ATP hydrolysis), minimize cellular perturbations, increase efficiency of motion, and improve the capacity of the trained musculature to resist fatigue (Hawley 2002). The mechanisms and metabolic signals by which active muscle senses homeostatic perturbations and then translates them into improved function has been a topic of intense research for several decades (for review, see Perry and Hawley 2017). It is now accepted that a variety of cellular disruptions takes place at the onset of exercise, including (but not limited to) increased cytoplasmic free $[Ca^{2+}]$, increased free AMP (AMPf) and an increased ADP/ATP ratio, reduced creatine phosphate and glycogen levels, increased FA concentrations and reactive oxygen/nitrogen species (ROS/RNS), acidosis and altered redox state, including [NAD/NADH] (Hawley et al. 2014; Perry and Hawley 2017). Within the context of metabolic homeostasis, an array of regulatory networks is stimulated that sustain rates of ATP synthesis over time through the activation of rate-limiting enzymes controlling carbohydrate and fat catabolism. A long-standing question in exercise biology is how do these acute disruptions in cellular signals that maintain energy supply also stimulate long-term adaptive processes that improve the ability of muscle to sustain a future contractile challenge?

A key component of improved "muscle fitness" following exercise training is biogenesis of mitochondria in skeletal muscle. A comprehensive discussion of this topic is beyond the scope of this chapter and the reader is referred to recent reviews (Hood et al. 2016; Perry and Hawley 2017). In brief, the molecular bases of skeletal muscle adaptations to an endurance exercise stimulus requires increased expression and/or activity of key mitochondrial proteins mediated by an array of intra-cellular signaling events, pre- and post-transcriptional processes, regulation of translation and protein expression, and modulation of protein (enzyme) activities and/or intra-cellular localization. There are multiple (and often redundant) stimuli associated with endurance exercise adaptations and numerous signaling kinases that respond to contractile stimuli, with numerous downstream pathways that are targets of these kinases (Egan et al. 2016; Hawley et al. 2014). A major advance in unraveling the cellular events that promote mitochondrial biogenesis was the discovery of the peroxisome-proliferator-activated receptor γ coactivator α (PGC-1α), an inducible coactivator that regulates the coordinated expression of mitochondrial proteins encoded in the nuclear and mitochondrial genomes (Lin et al. 2002). A critical feature of the PGC-1α coactivators is that they interact with many different transcription factors to activate distinct biological programs in several tissues (Lin et al. 2002). Certainly in skeletal muscle, PGC-1α has emerged as a key regulator of mitochondrial biogenesis responsive to the prevailing contractile activity.

The AMPK and p38 MAPK are two other important signaling cascades that converge upon the regulation of PGC-1α and consequently the regulation of mitochondrial biogenesis. The AMPK induces mitochondrial biogenesis partly by directly phosphorylating and activating PGC-1α (Jager et al. 2007) but also by phosphorylating the transcriptional repressor HDAC5, which relieves inhibition of the transcription factor myocyte enhancer factor 2 (MEF2), a known regulator of PGC-1α (McGee and Hargreaves 2010). p38 MAPK phosphorylates and activates PGC-1α (Puigserver et al. 2001) and also increases PGC-1α expression by phosphorylating the transcription factor ATF-2, which in turn increases PGC-1α protein abundance by binding to and activating the CREB site on the PGC-1α promoter (Akimoto et al. 2005). Another transcription factor involved in exercise-induced mitochondrial biogenesis in skeletal muscle and presumably activated by AMPK and/or p38 MAPK is the tumor suppressor protein p53. p53 knockout mice display reduced endurance exercise capacity compared with wild-type mice, along with reduced subsarcolemmal and inter-myofibrillar mitochondrial content and PGC-1α expression. p53 may also regulate exercise-induced mitochondrial biogenesis through interactions with TFAM in the mitochondria, where it functions to co-ordinate regulation of the mitochondrial genome (Saleem et al. 2011).

Train-Low, Compete High: A Novel Strategy to Augment Training Adaptation

Skeletal muscle glycogen availability exerts a regulatory effect on many cellular processes. As discussed, one protein with a fundamental role in monitoring cellular energy status is the AMPK. The recent discovery of glycogen-binding sites on the AMPK β-subunits (McBride et al. 2009) has led to the hypothesis that this regulatory domain may also allow AMPK to act as a sensor of endogenous glycogen stores (McBride and Hardie 2009). In this scenario, the glycogen-binding domains act as sensors, enabling AMPK to gauge the state of cellular glycogen, increasing AMPK activity when stores are low and decreasing the signal when stores are replete or elevated. The first experimental evidence from human skeletal muscle to provide indirect support for this hypothesis was undertaken by Wojtaszewski et al. (2003). These workers measured muscle-signaling responses and substrate utilization in well-trained males under conditions in which a standardized bout of exercise (1 h at 70% peak oxygen consumption) was commenced with either low (~160 mmol/kg dry wt) or high (~900 mmol/kg dry wt) muscle glycogen concentration. At rest, AMPK activity and acetyl-CoA carboxylase-β (ACC-β) Ser^{221}phosphorylation were lower in glycogen-loaded compared with glycogen-depleted muscles. Of note was the finding that concentrations of creatine phosphate and adenine nucleotides in resting muscles were similar despite large differences in muscle glycogen status, suggesting that fuel-dependent mechanisms independent of energy status might regulate AMPK signaling. AMPK-α1 and α2 activity and ACC-β Ser^{221} phosphorylation were activated to a greater extent when exercise was commenced with low compared to high glycogen levels. Subsequently, Steinberg et al. (2006) reported that commencing exercise with low muscle glycogen availability increased AMPK-α2 nuclear protein abundance. The results of these studies make it tempting to ascribe a direct mechanistic link between glycogen availability and AMPK activation. However, manipulating resting muscle glycogen content in humans also alters the concentrations of circulating blood metabolites (FFAs, catecholamines). These systemic factors are likely to "fine-tune" the signaling responses observed when exercise is commenced with low glycogen stores.

The early observations of increased AMPK activation when exercise is commenced with low muscle glycogen availability coupled with the putative role of the AMPK in many of the metabolic adaptations of skeletal muscle to exercise-training (Jørgensen et al. 2006; Pilegaard et al. 2002) were the bases of a hypothesis formulated by Hansen et al. (2005), namely that chronic exercise training undertaken with low muscle glycogen concentration would improve training adaptation to a greater extent compared to when all sessions were commenced with high glycogen availability. This training protocol was termed "train-low, compete-high." In a pioneering study, Hansen et al. (2005) used an experimental design in which the right and left legs of the same (untrained) subject performed the same amount of total work during a 10-week intervention period, albeit with different pre-exercise muscle glycogen content for half of the workouts. In agreement with their original hypothesis, they reported that markers of "training adaptation" (i.e., resting muscle glycogen content, the maximal activity of citrate synthase and performance time to exhaustion) were all enhanced to a greater extent in the leg that commenced selected training sessions with low compared with high muscle glycogen content (Hansen et al. 2005). The results of this study were groundbreaking, and the term "train-low, compete-high" rapidly spread among the athletic and scientific communities to describe this novel approach to training. However, the question of whether athletes with a history of endurance training would benefit to the same extent as previously untrained individuals when replacing a portion of their training program with "low glycogen" workouts could not be answered from the original study of Hansen et al. (2005).

In a follow-up investigation, Yeo et al. (2008) investigated the "train-low" paradigm during a 3-week intervention in well-trained endurance subjects: these researchers hypothesized that competitive athletes would have maximized their training adaptation, and further gains, even in the face of training-low, would be trivial. Yeo et al. (2008) imposed a training protocol in which nine intense interval-training sessions during the 3-week training block were commenced when glycogen stores were lowered by ~50% (through prior exercise) or were replete. Importantly, during these sessions, the work rate (power output, W) was not "clamped" as in the study of Hansen et al. (2005); rather athletes were asked to exercise as hard as they could and produce as much total work as possible. As expected, when athletes commenced training with low compared with normal glycogen availability, their maximal self-selected power output was significantly lower (an average of 7%). The remarkable finding, however, was that, despite a lower "training impulse" to the exercising musculature, resting muscle glycogen concentration, the maximal activities of citrate synthase and β-hydroxyacyl-CoA-dehydrogenase and the total protein content of cytochrome c oxidase subunit IV were higher (compared to pre-training values) in individuals who commenced interval training sessions with low muscle glycogen content. Despite these augmented training adaptations, which would be expected to enhance athletic performance, and in contrast to the findings of Hansen et al. (2005), there was no difference between the two treatment conditions in a sport-specific cycling time-trial (Yeo et al. (2008).

The precise mechanisms underlying an enhanced adaptive skeletal muscle response when training sessions were commenced with lowered glycogen availability were not investigated during these investigations (Hansen et al. 2005; Yeo et al. 2008). However, from earlier work, MAPK pathways have been implicated as possible signaling mechanisms involved in the regulation of exercise/nutrient adaptations. Chan et al. (2004) were the first to demonstrate that alterations in nutrient availability that reduced muscle glycogen content led to an increased phosphorylation of nuclear p38 MAPK in human skeletal muscle in response to moderate-intensity exercise. However, others have found little change in either the phosphorylation state of this kinase or one of its downstream targets (activating transcription factor 2) after a bout of intense cycling commenced with either low or normal muscle glycogen content (Yeo et al. 2010).

It is important to note that altering carbohydrate availability (i.e., lowering muscle glycogen content) has reciprocal and pronounced effects on lipid availability. Indeed it seems entirely plausible that increases in skeletal muscle mitochondria capacity could be further enhanced if training were performed under conditions that further elevated the levels of circulating FFAs. To test this hypothesis, Fillmore et al. (2010) determined whether a combination of chronic chemical activation of AMPK and high-fat availability (a low-CHO, high-fat diet) would have an additive effect on skeletal muscle mitochondria markers in a rodent model. They treated male Wistar rats with a high-fat diet, with injections of AICAR (an AMPK activator), or with a high-fat diet combined with AICAR injections for 6 weeks. Compared to either AICAR or high-fat feeding alone, AICAR treatment combined with high fat availability had an additive effect on markers of oxidative capacity (i.e., the citric acid cycle and electron transport chain) as well as transcriptional regulation. Specifically, long-chain acyl-CoA dehydrogenase, cytochrome c, PGC-1α protein, as well citrate synthase and β-hydroxyacyl-CoA dehydrogenase activity were all increased by a greater magnitude in the AICAR plus high-fat treatment. While the mechanism(s) responsible for the additive increase in mitochondrial content observed with chronic activation of AMPK and elevating circulating FFAs could not be directly determined, Fillmore et al. (2010) observed an synergistic effect of chronic AMPK activation and high-fat feeding on PGC-1α protein abundance and elevations in PGC-1α mRNA in response to chronic AMPK activation (but not by high-fat feeding). They concluded that the additive increase in PGC-1α protein abundance was a combined effect of high-fat feeding-induced posttranscriptional and AMPK-dependent transcriptional increases in PGC-1α protein expression. However, it should be noted that, when post- exercise increases in FA availability are abolished by administration of acipimox, a pharmacological inhibitor of lipolysis, the normal exercise-induced increase in mRNA abundance of selected metabolic genes (i.e., PDK4 and PGC-1α) persists (Tunstall et al. 2007). These data clearly demonstrate that the increase in circulating FFA concentrations observed during the later stages of exercise and subsequent recovery are not essential to induce skeletal muscle mRNA expression of several proteins involved in regulating muscle metabolism and training adaptation.

Evolution of a Paradigm: Train-High, Sleep-Low

The original "train low" protocol proposed by Hansen et al. (2005) and subsequently investigated by others (Hulston et al. 2010; Yeo et al. 2008) employed a twice-a-day training protocol in which the second exercise session was undertaken with low glycogen availability. As noted, a direct consequence of this strategy was that the maximal self-selected training intensity of the second session was substantially reduced when it was commenced with low compared with normal glycogen levels. Such an outcome is counter-intuitive for the preparation of competitive athletes for whom high-intensity workouts are a critical component of any periodized training program (Hawley and Burke 2010). Furthermore, it could be argued that training twice each day with workouts undertaken in close proximity underpinned part of the augmented training adaptation compared to once-a-day workouts. Against this background, we formulated a novel approach in which we can prolong the duration of low carbohydrate availability, thereby potentially enhancing and extending the time course of transcriptional activation of metabolic genes and their target proteins, while simultaneously conserving the training intensity of the initial session and hence the "training impulse" to the working muscles (Lane et al. 2015). We have termed this strategy "train-high, sleep-low." In this protocol, we periodized the timing of nutrient intake such that athletes performed an evening bout of high-intensity training with high carbohydrate availability, then restricted carbohydrate intake so that they slept with low carbohydrate availability before undertaking a prolonged exercise bout (120 min) in the fasted state the following morning. In our acute model (Lane et al. 2015), we found that, when feeding was withheld overnight and subjects slept with reduced carbohydrate availability, AMPKThr172, p38MAPK-Thr180/Tyr182, and p-ACCSer79 were upregulated to a greater extent the following morning, compared with when subjects were fed a high- carbohydrate meal the prior evening. We also showed that, when a second, prolonged steady-state training session was commenced after "sleeping low," the expression of selected genes and abundance of phosphorylated signaling proteins with putative roles in lipid oxidation and transport were higher compared with when a post-exercise meal was consumed and glycogen availability was partially restored (Lane et al. 2015). Importantly, subsequent chronic interventions utilizing the "train-high, sleep-low" approach over 1–3 weeks showed clear benefits to performance (Marquet et al. 2016a, b).

Summary and Directions for Future Research

Independent of prior training status, short-term (3- to 10-week) training programs in which some of the workouts are commenced with either low muscle glycogen availability (or low exogenous carbohydrate availability) augment training adaptation (i.e., they increase the maximal activities of selected enzymes involved in carbohydrate and/or lipid metabolism and promote mitochondrial biogenesis) to a greater extent than when all workouts are undertaken with normal or elevated glycogen stores. One aspect that is unclear from the present literature is the absolute levels of glycogen depletion needed to potentiate the effect of the training stimulus on outcomes such as mitochondrial biogenesis, or the length of time periodic low-glycogen training needs to be undertaken to demonstrate functional changes to training and/or performance outcomes. To answer such questions, a complex series of studies would need to be undertaken that systematically 'titrate' muscle glycogen levels and determine subsequent cellular (and performance) response to a standardized training regimen. A major problem for the basic scientist trying to unravel potential mechanism(s) underlying the benefit to training adaptation with reduced muscle glycogen availability is the fact that carbohydrate restriction has reciprocal and pronounced effects on lipid availability. To address this question, it will be necessary to study human subjects while they are consuming isoenergetic low carbohydrate diets in combination with either high protein or fat while undertaking a supervised exercise training protocol. Such experiments are currently being undertaken in our lab. Invasive measures of metabolism (i.e., markers of skeletal muscle mitochondrial biogenesis and respiration) are necessary to determine if it is high fat or low carbohydrate availability that drives the augmented training response. What is clear, however, is that in addition to their role as energy substrates, endogenous fuel stores and the concomitant changes in circulating hormones and metabolites can act as potent signaling intermediates to modify the normal responses to contractile activity, thereby augmenting training adaptation and ultimately driving some of the phenotypical changes observed with chronic exercise.

References

Akimoto T, Pohnert SC, Li P, Zhang M, Gumbs C, Rosenberg PB, Williams RS, Yan Z (2005) Exercise stimulates Pgc-1alpha transcription in skeletal muscle through activation of the p38 MAPK pathway. J Biol Chem 280:19587–19593

Bergström J, Hultman E (1966) Muscle glycogen synthesis after exercise: an enhancing factor localized to the muscle cells in man. Nature 210:309–310

Bonadonna RC, Groop LC, Zych K, Shank KM, DeFronzo RA (1990) Dose-dependent effect of insulin on plasma free fatty acid turnover and oxidation in humans. Am J Physiol Endocrinol Metab 259:E736–E750

Brooks GA, Mercier J (1994) Balance of carbohydrate and lipid utilization during exercise: the "crossover" concept. J Appl Physiol 76:2253–2261

Chan MH, McGee SL, Watt MJ, Hargreaves M, Febbraio MA (2004) Altering dietary nutrient intake that reduces glycogen content leads to phosphorylation of nuclear p38 MAP kinase in human skeletal muscle: association with IL-6 gene transcription during contraction. FASEB J 18:1785–1787

Coyle EF, Jeukendrup AE, Wagenmakers AJ, Saris WH (1997) Fatty acid oxidation is directly regulated by carbohydrate metabolism during exercise. Am J Physiol Endocrinol Metab 273:E268–E275

Egan B, Hawley JA, Zierath JR (2016) SnapShot: exercise metabolism. Cell Metab 24:342–342.e1

Fillmore N, Jacobs DL, Mills DB, Winder WW, Hancock CR (2010) Chronic AMP-activated protein kinase activation and a high-fat diet have an additive effect on mitochondria in rat skeletal muscle. J Appl Physiol 109:511–520

Galbo H, Holst JJ, Christensen NJ (1979) The effect of different diets and of insulin on the hormonal response to prolonged exercise. Acta Physiol Scand 107:19–32

Goldstein MS (1961) Humoral nature of the hypoglycemic factor of muscular work. Diabetes 10:232–234

Hansen AK, Fischer CP, Plomgaard P, Andersen JL, Saltin B, Pedersen BK (2005) Skeletal muscle adaptation: training twice every second day vs. training once daily. J Appl Physiol 98:93–99

Hawley JA (2002) Adaptations of skeletal muscle to prolonged, intense endurance training. Clin Exp Pharmacol Physiol 29:218–222

Hawley JA, Burke LM (2010) Carbohydrate availability and training adaptation: effects on cell metabolism. Exerc Sport Sci Rev 38:152–160

Hawley JA, Leckey JJ (2015) Carbohydrate dependence during prolonged, intense endurance exercise. Sports Med 45(Suppl 1):S5–12

Hawley JA, Hargreaves M, Joyner MJ, Zierath JR (2014) Integrative biology of exercise. Cell 159:738–749

Hawley JA, Maughan RJ, Hargreaves M (2015) Exercise metabolism: historical perspective. Cell Metab 22:12–17

Holloszy JO (1967) Biochemical adaptations in muscle. Effects of exercise on mitochondrial -oxygen uptake and respiratory enzyme activity in skeletal muscle. J Biol Chem 242:2278–2282

Holloszy JO, Kohrt WM, Hansen PA (1988) The regulation of carbohydrate and fat metabolism during and after exercise. Front Biosci 3:D1011–D1027

Hood DA, Tryon LD, Carter HN, Kim Y, Chen CC (2016) Unravelling the mechanisms regulating muscle mitochondrial biogenesis. Biochem J 473:2295–2314

Horowitz JF, Mora-Rodriguez R, Byerley LO, Coyle EF (1997) Lipolytic suppression following carbohydrate ingestion limits fat oxidation during exercise. Am J Physiol 273:E768–E775

Hulston CJ, Venables MC, Mann CH, Martin C, Philp A, Baar K, Jeukendrup AE (2010) Training with low muscle glycogen enhances fat metabolism in well-trained cyclists. Med Sci Sports Exerc 42:2046–2055

Jager S, Handschin C, St-Pierre J, Spiegelman BM (2007) AMP-activated protein kinase (AMPK) action in skeletal muscle via direct phosphorylation of PGC-1a. Proc Natl Acad Sci USA 104:12017–12022

Jørgensen SB, Richter EA, Wojtaszewski JFP (2006) Role of AMPK in skeletal muscle metabolic regulation and adaptation in relation to exercise. J Physiol 574:17–31

Lane SC, Camera DM, Lassiter DG, Areta JL, Bird SR, Yeo WK, Jeacocke NA, Krook A, Zierath JR, Burke LM, Hawley JA (2015) Effects of sleeping with reduced carbohydrate availability on acute training responses. J Appl Physiol 119:643–655

Lin J, Wu H, Tarr PT, Zhang CY, Wu Z, Boss O, Michael LF, Puigserver P, Isotani E, Olson EN, Lowell BB, Bassel-Duby R, Spiegelman BM (2002) Transcriptional co-activator PGC-1 alpha drives the formation of slow-twitch muscle fibres. Nature 418:797–801

Marquet LA, Brisswalter J, Louis J, Tiollier E, Burke LM, Hawley JA, Hausswirth C (2016a) Enhanced endurance performance by periodization of carbohydrate intake: "sleep low" strategy. Med Sci Sports Exerc 48:663–672

Marquet LA, Hausswirth C, Molle O, Hawley JA, Burke LM, Tiollier E, Brisswalter J (2016b) Periodization of carbohydrate intake: short-term effect on performance. Nutrients 8(12):E755

McBride A, Hardie DG (2009) AMP-activated protein kinase - a sensor of glycogen as well as AMP and ATP? Acta Physiol (Oxf) 196:99–113

McBride A, Ghilagaber S, Nikolaev A, Hardie DG (2009) The glycogen-binding domain on the AMPK beta subunit allows the kinase to act as a glycogen sensor. Cell Metab 9:23–34

McGee SL, Hargreaves M (2010) AMPK-mediated regulation of transcription in skeletal muscle. Clin Sci 118:507–518

Pedersen BK, Steensberg A, Fischer C, Keller C, Keller P, Plomgaard P, Febbraio M, Saltin B (2003) Searching for the exercise factor: is IL-6 a candidate? J Muscle Res Cell Motil 24:113–119

Perry CG, Hawley JA (2017) Molecular basis of exercise-induced skeletal muscle mitochondrial biogenesis: Historical advances, current knowledge, and future challenges. Cold Spring Harb Perspect Biol. pii: a029686

Perry CG, Lally J, Holloway GP, Heigenhauser GJ, Bonen A, Spriet LL (2010) Repeated transient mRNA bursts precede increases in transcriptional and mitochondrial proteins during training in human skeletal muscle. J Physiol 588:4795–4810

Pilegaard H, Keller C, Steensberg A, Helge JW, Pedersen BK, Saltin B, Neufer PD (2002) Influence of pre-exercise muscle glycogen content on exercise-induced transcriptional regulation of metabolic genes. J Physiol 541:261–271

Puigserver P, Rhee J, Lin J, Wu Z, Yoon JC, Zhang CY, Krauss S, Mootha VK, Lowell BB, Spiegelman BM (2001) Cytokine stimulation of energy expenditure through p38 MAP kinase activation of PPARgamma coactivator-1. Mol Cell 8:971–982

Randle PJ (1986) Fuel selection in animals. Biochem Soc Trans 14:799–806

Randle PJ, Newsholme EA, Garland PB (1964) Regulation of glucose uptake by muscle. 8. Effects of fatty acids, ketone bodies and pyruvate, and of alloxan-diabetes and starvation, on the uptake and metabolic fate of glucose in rat heart and diaphragm muscles. Biochem J 93:652–665

Romijn JA, Coyle EF, Sidossis LS, Zhang XJ, Wolfe RR (1995) Relationship between fatty acid delivery and fatty acid oxidation during strenuous exercise. J Appl Physiol 79:1939–1945

Saleem A, Carter HN, Iqbal S, Hood DA (2011) Role of p53 within the regulatory network controlling muscle mitochondrial biogenesis. Exerc Sport Sci Rev 39:199–205

Steinberg GR, Watt MJ, McGee SL, Chan S, Hargreaves M, Febbraio MA, Stapleton D, Kemp BE (2006) Reduced glycogen availability is associated with increased AMPKalpha2 activity, nuclear AMPKalpha2 protein abundance, and GLUT4 mRNA expression in contracting human skeletal muscle. Appl Physiol Nutr Metab 31:302–312

Tunstall RJ, McAinch AJ, Hargreaves M, van Loon LJ, Cameron-Smith D (2007) Reduced plasma free fatty acid availability during exercise: effect on gene expression. Eur J Appl Physiol 99:485–493

Wojtaszewski JF, MacDonald C, Nielsen JN, Hellsten Y, Hardie DG, Kemp BE, Kiens B, Richter EA (2003) Regulation of 5'AMP-activated protein kinase activity and substrate utilization in exercising human skeletal muscle. Am J Physiol Endocrinol Metab 284:E813–E822

Yeo WK, Paton CD, Garnham AP, Burke LM, Carey AL, Hawley JA (2008) Skeletal muscle adaptation and performance responses to once a day versus twice every second day endurance training regimens. J Appl Physiol 105:1462–1470
Yeo WK, McGee SL, Carey AL, Paton CD, Garnham AP, Hargreaves M, Hawley JA (2010) Acute signalling responses to intense endurance training commenced with low or normal muscle glycogen. Exp Physiol 95:351–358

Optimized Engagement of Macrophages and Satellite Cells in the Repair and Regeneration of Exercised Muscle

Check for updates

Regula Furrer and Christoph Handschin

Abstract Recurring contraction-relaxation cycles exert a massive mechanical load on muscle fibers. Training adaptation therefore entails the promotion of a series of biological programs aimed at inducing a better stress response but also at optimizing repair processes. Muscle regeneration is controlled by an intricate, tightly coordinated engagement of muscle fibers, satellite cells, macrophages and other cell types. In this review, we discuss some of the recent insights into the regulation of muscle repair and regeneration in exercised muscle, elucidate the role of the peroxisome proliferator-activated receptor γ coactivator 1α (PGC-1α) in this context, and speculate about potential implications for the treatment of muscle diseases.

Introduction

Skeletal muscle is a highly plastic organ that adapts its properties depending on contractile demand. These adaptations are not only affected by mechanical loading, e.g., as seen after a period of inactivity or training, but also by the availability of nutrients and hormones, temperature or oxygen levels, which collectively determine the balance between protein synthesis and degradation, mitochondrial activity, contractile function, a shift in fiber type distribution and other biological programs. For example, endurance training promotes mitochondrial function and oxidative metabolism, a shift towards high endurance muscle fibers and tissue vascularization, among other changes. The peroxisome proliferator-activated receptor γ coactivator 1α (PGC-1α) is an important driver of endurance training adaptation (Lin et al. 2002, 2005; Handschin 2010). Accordingly, PGC-1α strongly boosts oxidative metabolism, a fiber type shift, glucose uptake, vascularization and other properties of endurance-trained fibers by co-activating a variety of transcription factors in a complex transcriptional network (Handschin 2010; Kupr and Handschin 2015).

R. Furrer • C. Handschin (✉)
Biozentrum, University of Basel, Basel, Switzerland
e-mail: christoph.handschin@unibas.ch

© The Author(s) 2017
B. Spiegelman (ed.), *Hormones, Metabolism and the Benefits of Exercise*,
Research and Perspectives in Endocrine Interactions,
https://doi.org/10.1007/978-3-319-72790-5_5

Exercise is one of the best interventions to preserve muscle mass through its strong anti-atrophic effects. As one of the main effectors of exercise adaptation, PGC-1α also reduces the pathological consequences of muscle wasting. For example, elevation of PGC-1α in skeletal muscle reduces fiber damage and atrophy and improves muscle functionality in etiologically diverse muscle wasting contexts such as hind limb unloading (Cannavino et al. 2014), denervation or fasting (Sandri et al. 2006), or even Duchenne muscular dystrophy (DMD; Handschin et al. 2007; Selsby et al. 2012; Hollinger et al. 2013). Several mechanisms have been proposed to be involved in the therapeutic effect of PGC-1α in muscle pathologies, for example, the inhibition of the transcriptional activity of forkhead box O3 (FoxO3) and thereby the induction of E3 ubiquitin ligases muscle ring finger 1 (MuRF-1) and muscle atrophy f-box (MAFbx) that promote protein degradation and fiber atrophy (Sandri et al. 2006). However, other consequences of increased PGC-1α activity have also been implicated; therefore, the exact mechanisms that underlie the beneficial effect of elevation of PGC-1α remain unclear. More recently, the involvement of inflammation, both in muscle fibers and through activation of resident macrophages and satellite cells (SCs), the lineage-committed adult muscle stem cells, has been studied in more detail in this context.

Repair and Regeneration After Muscle Damage

For proper muscle regeneration, a series of highly coordinated events take place that entail a tightly orchestrated cross-talk between different cell types to ensure proper initiation, activation, cell type transition and, ultimately, termination of various cellular programs. Initially, in response to injury, muscle cells and tissue-resident macrophages secrete cytokines and chemokines such as tumor necrosis factor α (TNFα) and C-C motif ligand 2/monocyte chemoattractant protein-1 (CCL2/MCP-1) to attract additional immune cells (Pillon et al. 2013). Neutrophils are among the first leukocytes infiltrating the damaged area, and they subsequently release chemotactic signals to promote the tissue infiltration by circulating monocytes (Saclier et al. 2013a). During the initial inflammatory response, monocytes polarize into classical M1-type-activated macrophages and remove tissue debris by phagocytosis. The concomitantly secreted cytokine and chemokine cocktail not only further attracts monocytes but also activates SC proliferation and commitment (Saclier et al. 2013b). The SCs are located in the niche between the sarcolemma and the basal lamina and express different factors depending on the state of the myogenic process. Quiescent SCs are characterized by high levels of paired-box 7 (Pax7). Upon activation, e.g., by muscle injury, proliferation and commitment are initiated by a switch to myogenic regulatory factor 5 (Myf5) and MyoD expression, ultimately resulting in the differentiation into myoblasts and subsequent fusion to myofibers with elevated myogenin and MRF4 (Charge and Rudnicki 2004). This differentiation process is promoted by the shift in macrophage polarization into the alternatively activated M2 types that release anti-inflammatory factors (Saclier et al. 2013b). The requirement for a tight orchestration of these different phases is illustrated, for example, by the fibrotic tissue accumulation in the case of a disruption of the regeneration process by a prolongation of the initial pro-inflammatory context, thereby resulting in impaired muscle function. Inversely, a reduced phase involving M1 macrophages may impair regeneration by increased formation of necrotic tissue and inhibition of proliferation of myogenic cells. Therefore, the tight coordination of the transition from M1 to M2 macrophages is critical for proper regeneration.

Effects of Exercise and PGC-1α on SCs

In several pathological conditions such as DMD, cancer cachexia and aging, oxidative muscle fibers are preferentially spared, suggesting that these muscle fibers are more protected from muscle damage and degradation. Interestingly, the SC pool in highly oxidative muscle fibers is larger (Gibson and Schultz 1982; Dinulovic et al. 2016b), which could contribute to an improved regeneration after muscle damage. Therefore, inducing a shift towards an oxidative phenotype of the muscle by, for example, exercise (Rowe et al. 2014a), which is also accompanied by a higher SC content (Shefer et al. 2010; Kurosaka et al. 2012; Fry et al. 2014; Abreu et al. 2017), could be a strategy to ameliorate the progression of these pathologies. Even in old muscle, the aging-induced loss of SCs and differentiation potential can be preserved by voluntary wheel running or forced treadmill exercise by increased Wnt signaling (Fujimaki et al. 2014; Cisterna et al. 2016). The rejuvenating effect of exercise on SC function was demonstrated in aged trained mice that recovered to a similar extent as young sedentary animals after muscle injury (Joanisse et al. 2016), indicating that the reduced regenerative capacity of aging muscles could be restored by exercise.

Curiously, even though many of the exercise-induced adaptations in muscle, such as the fiber type shift and oxidative metabolism, are regulated by PGC-1α (Lin et al. 2002, 2005; Handschin 2010); the number of SCs in mice overexpressing PGC-1α specifically in muscle (MCKα) is lower than in wild-type animals and thus diametrically opposite to the higher number seen after exercise or in oxidative muscles (Dinulovic et al. 2016b). Importantly however, despite the reduced SC pool, regeneration is not impaired and the proliferative potential of the SCs is even enhanced in these mice (Dinulovic et al. 2016b). These observations suggest that PGC-1α indirectly affects SC function by co-activating factors that activate SCs or induce a change in the SC niche (Fig. 1).

The composition of the extracellular matrix (ECM) and the basal lamina determines the efficacy of the niche to modulate SC proliferation and differentiation. For example, fibronectin (FN) is an important niche protein involved in the activation and proliferation of SCs (Bentzinger et al. 2013). Accordingly, the impaired regenerative capacity in aging muscle is associated with reduced levels of FN and can be restored by treating mice with FN (Lukjanenko et al. 2016). It is conceivable,

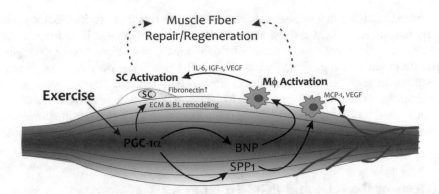

Fig. 1 Pre-conditioning of the muscle for faster regeneration. Schematic representation of the exercise- and PGC-1α-induced muscle cross-talk to macrophages and satellite cells (SC) that creates an environment that could prime the tissue for improved regeneration in response to damage. *ECM* extracellular matrix, *BL* basal lamina, *Mφ* Macrophage

therefore, that the enhanced proliferative potential of SCs of MCKα mice is linked to FN function, since higher levels of FN are observed in the muscles of these animals (Dinulovic et al. 2016b). The increase in matrix metalloproteinases 2 (MMP2) and MMP9 induced by exercise further underscores the importance of niche remodeling, since the ensuing ECM degradation could subsequently facilitate the migration of SCs (Garg and Boppart 2016) whereas MMP-controlled vascularization enhances the delivery of nutrients and growth factors to the niche (Gustafsson 2011). Accordingly, differentiating SCs are closer to capillaries compared to quiescent SCs (Christov et al. 2007). Inversely, SCs are more distantly located from capillaries in old compared to young men (Nederveen et al. 2016), suggesting that the reduced transport of signaling molecules to the niche could contribute to the reduced regenerating potential observed in aging muscles. The angiogenesis induced by exercise or PGC-1α (Gustafsson 2011; Rowe et al. 2014b) results in a closer proximity of SCs to capillaries; hence there is improved transport of circulating factors to the niche and ultimately enhanced regenerative processes.

Effects of Exercise and PGC-1α on Macrophages and Inflammation

In contrast to the numerous studies on the effects of exercise on SCs, literature on exercise-induced changes on macrophages is scarce. Most studies investigating macrophage infiltration in the context of regeneration post-exercise were performed in humans after damaging eccentric exercise (Przybyla et al. 2006; Mahoney et al. 2008; MacNeil et al. 2011), and less is known about the effects of endurance exercise on macrophage infiltration. As infiltration of immune cells is tightly coordinated, the timing of tissue collection is crucial and complicates the experimental setup. In response to resistance exercise, infiltration of CD68[+] macrophages is increased after 48 h (Mahoney et al. 2008; MacNeil et al. 2011) and unchanged in the early (3 h) and late (72 h) phases of recovery (Przybyla et al. 2006; Mahoney et al. 2008; MacNeil et al. 2011). The expected switch to CD163[+] M2 macrophages is observed after 72 h, i.e., during the later stage of regeneration (Przybyla et al. 2006). In contrast to the infiltration of macrophages seen 48 h post-resistance exercise in humans, endurance exercise had no effect on the number of macrophages at that time point in rats (Kurosaka et al. 2012). Therefore, the timing of macrophage activation, infiltration and polarization depends on the type of exercise, training intensity and most likely other factors that remain to be elucidated.

In skeletal muscle fibers, PGC-1α reduces the expression of pro-inflammatory gene expression by inhibiting the transcriptional activity of the nuclear factor κB (NF-κB; Eisele et al. 2013). Nevertheless, somewhat unexpectedly, sustained over-expression of PGC-1α in muscle increases the number of tissue-resident macrophages in uninjured muscle (Rowe et al. 2014b; Dinulovic et al. 2016a). However, these macrophages have a predominant M2 phenotype (Dinulovic et al. 2016a), indicating that PGC-1α induces an anti-inflammatory environment and may thereby modulate the response to muscle damage. Interestingly, in contrast to the glycolytic phenotype of M1 macrophages, M2 macrophages have a more oxidative phenotype (Galvan-Pena and O'Neill 2014; Kelly and O'Neill 2015), analogous to the metabolic phenotype of muscle overexpressing PGC-1α or PGC-1β. The metabolic shift required for the anti-inflammatory phenotype of macrophages is mediated by PGC-1β (Vats et al. 2006).

Although the mechanisms by which PGC-1α affects macrophage polarization leading to the higher number of M2 macrophages in muscle is unknown, mediators of PGC-1α-dependent macrophage attraction and/or activation have been described (Fig. 1). PGC-1α induces the transcription of secreted phosphoprotein 1 (SPP1), which in turn is involved in the recruitment of macrophages and activation of epithelial cells to ensure functional neovascularization (Rowe et al. 2014b). In the context of acute exercise, PGC-1α controls the expression of the B-type natriuretic peptide (BNP), which promotes macrophage activation in a paracrine manner (Furrer et al. 2017). While M1 macrophage activation is resolved more rapidly in damaged PGC-1α-overexpressing muscles (Dinulovic et al. 2016a), the mechanisms by which muscle PGC-1α affects infiltration and polarization in this context are still unclear.

Exercise-Induced Pre-conditioning for Faster Muscle Regeneration

As described above, exercise and muscle PGC-1α induce several adaptations such as an increase in the SC pool, remodeling of the SC niche, enhancement of the proliferation and differentiation potential of SCs as well as a higher number of tissue-resident macrophages that could all contribute to an improved regenerative capacity of the muscle. It is conceivable that exercise creates an environment within the muscle and the niche that could prime the muscle for improved regeneration in response to muscle damage. This hypothesis of exercise-induced pre-conditioning is supported by various observations. For example, the altered tissue-resident macrophage population in muscles overexpressing PGC-1α could contribute to the improved SC proliferation and commitment in damaged muscles of these mice, since a variety of cytokines and growth factors that activate SCs are secreted by both muscle and macrophages. M1 macrophages release interleukin 6 (IL-6), insulin-like growth factor 1 (IGF-1) and vascular endothelial growth factor (VEGF), whereas M2 macrophages mainly secrete IGF-1 and VEGF (Wu et al. 2010; Lu et al. 2011; Tonkin et al. 2015). IL-6 and IGF-1 are important for the activation and proliferation of SC (Charge and Rudnicki 2004; Serrano et al. 2008) and may thereby contribute not only to the repair and regeneration but, in the case of resistance training, also the hypertrophic response to exercise. Besides the direct effect of IL-6 on SCs, changes in IL-6 levels may also be involved in the remodeling of the niche, as IL-6 KO mice show lower levels of FN (Serrano et al. 2008). These reduced FN levels contribute to impaired regeneration, which is in line with the FN-dependent decrease in regeneration observed in aging (Lukjanenko et al. 2016). Therefore, the number of macrophages as well as the proportion of M1 and M2 macrophages in a trained muscle could play a role in the pre-conditioning of the muscle.

Of note, several of these factors, such as IL-6, IGF-1 and VEGF, are also myokines that are produced and secreted from muscle after exercise (Schnyder and Handschin 2015). Collectively, the local levels of such signaling molecules could, therefore, affect the activation of both macrophages and SCs. For example, elevation of VEGF stimulates angiogenesis and thereby increases vascularization (Gustafsson 2011; Rowe et al. 2014b). The increase in VEGF is directly regulated by PGC-1α in muscle fibers (Arany et al. 2008; Baresic et al. 2014; Rowe et al. 2014b) and potentially also indirectly through the stimulation of M2 macrophage accumulation (Dinulovic et al. 2016a). The resulting increase in tissue vascularization improves activation of SCs and facilitates infiltration of immune cells.

Besides paracrine effects of muscle and macrophages, exercise-regulated modulation of intrinsic SC properties also influences the proliferation and differentiation potential. For example, isolated SCs of muscles exposed to functional overload fuse better than control SCs (Fujimaki et al. 2016), suggesting that the differentiation potential of SCs is improved by exercise in a manner that is maintained even after removal from the niche. Inactivation of Notch signaling and stimulation of Wnt signaling contribute to improved fusion of trained SCs (Fujimaki et al. 2016), but the exact mechanisms of this priming of SC memory is unclear. Recently, a G_{0alert} state of SCs in the contralateral, non-damaged leg of mice with a pharmacologically induced muscle injury has been proposed to be linked to mammalian target of rapamycin complex 1 (mTORC1) activity (Rodgers et al. 2014). This SC pool exhibits an accelerated proliferative response upon activation. Similar to these observations in SCs, muscles may also have a memory in terms of the post-exercise inflammatory response: in human volunteers, MCP-1 levels as well as CD68[+]

macrophages were higher two days after a repeated bout compared to the first bout of exercise (Deyhle et al. 2015). While the mechanisms underlying this finding remain enigmatic, similar exacerbated macrophage activation is observed upon elevation of BNP by PGC-1α in exercised muscle (Furrer et al. 2017). Moreover, in muscles overexpressing PGC-1α, a larger area of cardiotoxin-damaged muscle is covered by macrophages and thus undergoing regeneration (Dinulovic et al. 2016a). In addition, after chronic muscle damage by multiple cardiotoxin injections, fiber size was recovered more efficiently and fibrotic tissue was reduced by PGC-1α overexpression (Dinulovic et al. 2016a, b), indicating that exercise- and PGC-1α-induced intrinsic and extrinsic adaptations contributed to enhanced regenerative capacity. Importantly, improved regeneration upon cardiotoxin-induced muscle damage occurred despite strong downregulation of PGC-1α expression (Dinulovic et al. 2016a, b). These data strongly imply a pre-conditioning effect to help trained muscle to cope with damage that includes a broad spectrum of functional modulation of SCs, endothelial cells and macrophages as well as cellular cross-talk that together create an environment that primes the muscle for faster regeneration.

Conclusion

Overexpression of PGC-1α in skeletal muscle ameliorates the symptoms of many different muscle diseases. Similarly, in those pathologies in which patients are exercise tolerant, training confers a beneficial effect on muscle functionality. While many different properties of exercise and PGC-1α most likely contribute to this therapeutic effect, the modulation and orchestration of macrophages and SCs could directly improve repair and regeneration in these diseases. Therefore, a more careful elucidation of the cell autonomous changes and cellular cross-talk that optimize repair and regeneration of damaged muscle tissue after exercise could provide novel targets and avenues to treat a wide variety of different muscle diseases.

Acknowledgments The work in our group related to the topic of this review is supported by the Swiss National Science Foundation, the European Research Council (ERC) Consolidator grant 616830 MUSCLE_NET, Swiss Cancer Research grant KFS-3733-08-2015, the Swiss Society for Research on Muscle Diseases (SSEM), SystemsX.ch and the University of Basel.

References

Abreu P, Mendes SV, Ceccatto VM, Hirabara SM (2017) Satellite cell activation induced by aerobic muscle adaptation in response to endurance exercise in humans and rodents. Life Sci 170:33–40

Arany Z, Foo SY, Ma Y, Ruas JL, Bommi-Reddy A, Girnun G, Cooper M, Laznik D, Chinsomboon J, Rangwala SM, Baek KH, Rosenzweig A, Spiegelman BM (2008) HIF-independent regulation of VEGF and angiogenesis by the transcriptional coactivator PGC-1alpha. Nature 451:1008–1012

Baresic M, Salatino S, Kupr B, van Nimwegen E, Handschin C (2014) Transcriptional network analysis in muscle reveals AP-1 as a partner of PGC-1alpha in the regulation of the hypoxic gene program. Mol Cell Biol 34:2996–3012

Bentzinger CF, Wang YX, von Maltzahn J, Soleimani VD, Yin H, Rudnicki MA (2013) Fibronectin regulates Wnt7a signaling and satellite cell expansion. Cell Stem Cell 12:75–87

Cannavino J, Brocca L, Sandri M, Bottinelli R, Pellegrino MA (2014) PGC1-alpha over-expression prevents metabolic alterations and soleus muscle atrophy in hindlimb unloaded mice. J Physiol 592:4575–4589

Charge SB, Rudnicki MA (2004) Cellular and molecular regulation of muscle regeneration. Physiol Rev 84:209–238

Christov C, Chretien F, Abou-Khalil R, Bassez G, Vallet G, Authier FJ, Bassaglia Y, Shinin V, Tajbakhsh S, Chazaud B, Gherardi RK (2007) Muscle satellite cells and endothelial cells: close neighbors and privileged partners. Mol Biol Cell 18:1397–1409

Cisterna B, Giagnacovo M, Costanzo M, Fattoretti P, Zancanaro C, Pellicciari C, Malatesta M (2016) Adapted physical exercise enhances activation and differentiation potential of satellite cells in the skeletal muscle of old mice. J Anat 228:771–783

Deyhle MR, Gier AM, Evans KC, Eggett DL, Nelson WB, Parcell AC, Hyldahl RD (2015) Skeletal muscle inflammation following repeated bouts of lengthening contractions in humans. Front Physiol 6:424

Dinulovic I, Furrer R, Di Fulvio S, Ferry A, Beer M, Handschin C (2016a) PGC-1alpha modulates necrosis, inflammatory response, and fibrotic tissue formation in injured skeletal muscle. Skelet Muscle 6:38

Dinulovic I, Furrer R, Beer M, Ferry A, Cardel B, Handschin C (2016b) Muscle PGC-1α modulates satellite cell number and proliferation by remodeling the stem cell niche. Skelet Muscle 6:39

Eisele PS, Salatino S, Sobek J, Hottiger MO, Handschin C (2013) The peroxisome proliferator-activated receptor gamma coactivator 1alpha/beta (PGC-1) coactivators repress the transcriptional activity of NF-kappaB in skeletal muscle cells. J Biol Chem 288:2246–2260

Fry CS, Noehren B, Mula J, Ubele MF, Westgate PM, Kern PA, Peterson CA (2014) Fibre type-specific satellite cell response to aerobic training in sedentary adults. J Physiol 592:2625–2635

Fujimaki S, Hidaka R, Asashima M, Takemasa T, Kuwabara T (2014) Wnt protein-mediated satellite cell conversion in adult and aged mice following voluntary wheel running. J Biol Chem 289:7399–7412

Fujimaki S, Machida M, Wakabayashi T, Asashima M, Takemasa T, Kuwabara T (2016) Functional overload enhances satellite cell properties in skeletal muscle. Stem Cells Int 2016:7619418

Furrer R, Eisele PS, Schmidt A, Beer M, Handschin C (2017) Paracrine cross-talk between skeletal muscle and macrophages in exercise by PGC-1α-controlled BNP. Sci Rep 7:40789

Galvan-Pena S, O'Neill LA (2014) Metabolic reprograming in macrophage polarization. Front Immunol 5:420

Garg K, Boppart MD (2016) Influence of exercise and aging on extracellular matrix composition in the skeletal muscle stem cell niche. J Appl Physiol (1985) 121:1053–1058

Gibson MC, Schultz E (1982) The distribution of satellite cells and their relationship to specific fiber types in soleus and extensor digitorum longus muscles. Anat Rec 202:329–337

Gustafsson T (2011) Vascular remodelling in human skeletal muscle. Biochem Soc Trans 39:1628–1632

Handschin C (2010) Regulation of skeletal muscle cell plasticity by the peroxisome proliferator-activated receptor gamma coactivator 1alpha. J Recept Signal Transduct Res 30:376–384

Handschin C, Kobayashi YM, Chin S, Seale P, Campbell KP, Spiegelman BM (2007) PGC-1alpha regulates the neuromuscular junction program and ameliorates Duchenne muscular dystrophy. Genes Dev 21:770–783

Hollinger K, Gardan-Salmon D, Santana C, Rice D, Snella E, Selsby JT (2013) Rescue of dystrophic skeletal muscle by PGC-1alpha involves restored expression of dystrophin-associated protein complex components and satellite cell signaling. Am J Physiol Regul Integr Comp Physiol 305:R13–R23

Joanisse S, Nederveen JP, Baker JM, Snijders T, Iacono C, Parise G (2016) Exercise conditioning in old mice improves skeletal muscle regeneration. FASEB J 30:3256–3268

Kelly B, O'Neill LA (2015) Metabolic reprogramming in macrophages and dendritic cells in innate immunity. Cell Res 25:771–784

Kupr B, Handschin C (2015) Complex coordination of cell plasticity by a PGC-1alpha-controlled transcriptional network in skeletal muscle. Front Physiol 6:325

Kurosaka M, Naito H, Ogura Y, Machida S, Katamoto S (2012) Satellite cell pool enhancement in rat plantaris muscle by endurance training depends on intensity rather than duration. Acta Physiol (Oxf) 205:159–166

Lin J, Wu H, Tarr PT, Zhang CY, Wu Z, Boss O, Michael LF, Puigserver P, Isotani E, Olson EN, Lowell BB, Bassel-Duby R, Spiegelman BM (2002) Transcriptional co-activator PGC-1 alpha drives the formation of slow-twitch muscle fibres. Nature 418:797–801

Lin J, Handschin C, Spiegelman BM (2005) Metabolic control through the PGC-1 family of transcription coactivators. Cell Metab 1:361–370

Lu H, Huang D, Saederup N, Charo IF, Ransohoff RM, Zhou L (2011) Macrophages recruited via CCR2 produce insulin-like growth factor-1 to repair acute skeletal muscle injury. FASEB J 25:358–369

Lukjanenko L et al (2016) Loss of fibronectin from the aged stem cell niche affects the regenerative capacity of skeletal muscle in mice. Nat Med 22:897–905

MacNeil LG, Baker SK, Stevic I, Tarnopolsky MA (2011) 17beta-estradiol attenuates exercise-induced neutrophil infiltration in men. Am J Physiol Regul Integr Comp Physiol 300:R1443–R1451

Mahoney DJ, Safdar A, Parise G, Melov S, Fu M, MacNeil L, Kaczor J, Payne ET, Tarnopolsky MA (2008) Gene expression profiling in human skeletal muscle during recovery from eccentric exercise. Am J Physiol Regul Integr Comp Physiol 294:R1901–R1910

Nederveen JP, Joanisse S, Snijders T, Ivankovic V, Baker SK, Phillips SM, Parise G (2016) Skeletal muscle satellite cells are located at a closer proximity to capillaries in healthy young compared with older men. J Cachexia Sarcopenia Muscle 7:547–554

Pillon NJ, Bilan PJ, Fink LN, Klip A (2013) Cross-talk between skeletal muscle and immune cells: muscle-derived mediators and metabolic implications. Am J Physiol Endocrinol Metab 304:E453–E465

Przybyla B, Gurley C, Harvey JF, Bearden E, Kortebein P, Evans WJ, Sullivan DH, Peterson CA, Dennis RA (2006) Aging alters macrophage properties in human skeletal muscle both at rest and in response to acute resistance exercise. Exp Gerontol 41:320–327

Rodgers JT, King KY, Brett JO, Cromie MJ, Charville GW, Maguire KK, Brunson C, Mastey N, Liu L, Tsai CR, Goodell MA, Rando TA (2014) mTORC1 controls the adaptive transition of quiescent stem cells from G(0) to G(Alert). Nature 510:393–396

Rowe GC, Safdar A, Arany Z (2014a) Running forward: new frontiers in endurance exercise biology. Circulation 129:798–810

Rowe GC, Raghuram S, Jang C, Nagy JA, Patten IS, Goyal A, Chan MC, Liu LX, Jiang A, Spokes KC, Beeler D, Dvorak H, Aird WC, Arany Z (2014b) PGC-1alpha induces SPP1 to activate macrophages and orchestrate functional angiogenesis in skeletal muscle. Circ Res 115:504–517

Saclier M, Cuvellier S, Magnan M, Mounier R, Chazaud B (2013a) Monocyte/macrophage interactions with myogenic precursor cells during skeletal muscle regeneration. FEBS J 280:4118–4130

Saclier M, Yacoub-Youssef H, Mackey AL, Arnold L, Ardjoune H, Magnan M, Sailhan F, Chelly J, Pavlath GK, Mounier R, Kjaer M, Chazaud B (2013b) Differentially activated macrophages orchestrate myogenic precursor cell fate during human skeletal muscle regeneration. Stem Cells 31:384–396

Sandri M, Lin J, Handschin C, Yang W, Arany ZP, Lecker SH, Goldberg AL, Spiegelman BM (2006) PGC-1alpha protects skeletal muscle from atrophy by suppressing FoxO3 action and atrophy-specific gene transcription. Proc Natl Acad Sci USA 103:16260–16265

Schnyder S, Handschin C (2015) Skeletal muscle as an endocrine organ: PGC-1alpha, myokines and exercise. Bone 80:115–125

Selsby JT, Morine KJ, Pendrak K, Barton ER, Sweeney HL (2012) Rescue of dystrophic skeletal muscle by PGC-1alpha involves a fast to slow fiber type shift in the mdx mouse. PLoS One 7:e30063

Serrano AL, Baeza-Raja B, Perdiguero E, Jardi M, Munoz-Canoves P (2008) Interleukin-6 is an essential regulator of satellite cell-mediated skeletal muscle hypertrophy. Cell Metab 7:33–44

Shefer G, Rauner G, Yablonka-Reuveni Z, Benayahu D (2010) Reduced satellite cell numbers and myogenic capacity in aging can be alleviated by endurance exercise. PLoS One 5:e13307

Tonkin J, Temmerman L, Sampson RD, Gallego-Colon E, Barberi L, Bilbao D, Schneider MD, Musaro A, Rosenthal N (2015) Monocyte/macrophage-derived IGF-1 orchestrates murine skeletal muscle regeneration and modulates autocrine polarization. Mol Ther 23:1189–1200

Vats D, Mukundan L, Odegaard JI, Zhang L, Smith KL, Morel CR, Wagner RA, Greaves DR, Murray PJ, Chawla A (2006) Oxidative metabolism and PGC-1beta attenuate macrophage-mediated inflammation. Cell Metab 4:13–24

Wu WK, Llewellyn OP, Bates DO, Nicholson LB, Dick AD (2010) IL-10 regulation of macrophage VEGF production is dependent on macrophage polarisation and hypoxia. Immunobiology 215:796–803

Skeletal Muscle microRNAs: Roles in Differentiation, Disease and Exercise

Rasmus J. O. Sjögren, Magnus H. L. Lindgren Niss, and Anna Krook

Abstract MicroRNAs (miRNA) are a noncoding RNA species that play important roles in the regulation of gene expression. Since miRNAs are able to target multiple genes simultaneously, miRNAs provide a mechanism for efficiently modulating a whole pathway to change or alter the functional properties in a particular target tissue. Ablation of miRNA processing specifically in skeletal muscle results in muscle abnormalities and perinatal death, underscoring that miRNAs control essential processes in skeletal muscle development and function. In this chapter we summarise current knowledge on miRNAs involved in skeletal muscle differentiation, disease and exercise.

Discovery and Biological Role of miRNAs

Precise control of gene expression and hence transcriptional regulation is a prerequisite for maintaining cellular functions, including growth and metabolic homeostasis. Several epigenetic factors, including DNA methylation, histone modification and miRNAs play important roles in gene expression in multicellular organisms. miRNAs were first described at the beginning of the 1990s, when it was appreciated that these short single-stranded non-coding RNAs function to post-transcriptionally regulate mRNA abundance and protein translation. Lin-4 and let-7 were the first miRNAs to be identified and found to be involved in the regulation of larval development of *C. elegans* (Lee et al. 1993; Wightman et al. 1993; Reinhart et al. 2000). miRNAs have since been observed in viruses, plants and mammals (Bartel 2009) and found to regulate a wide variety of cellular functions, including proliferation, differentiation and metabolism (He et al. 2007b; Williams et al. 2009a; Massart et al. 2016).

R. J. O. Sjögren
Department of Molecular Medicine and Surgery, Karolinska Institutet, Stockholm, Sweden

M. H. L. Lindgren Niss • A. Krook (✉)
Department of Physiology and Pharmacology, Integrative Physiology, Karolinska Institutet, Stockholm, Sweden
e-mail: anna.krook@ki.se

© The Author(s) 2017
B. Spiegelman (ed.), *Hormones, Metabolism and the Benefits of Exercise*,
Research and Perspectives in Endocrine Interactions,
https://doi.org/10.1007/978-3-319-72790-5_6

miRNA Biogenesis, mRNA Interaction and Target Prediction

miRNAs are expressed in the nucleus as primary-miRNA (pri-miRNA) transcripts, which require processing before becoming functional miRNAs. Pri-miRNAs contain stem-loop structures that are recognized and cleaved by the RNase III endonuclease Drosha to form precursor miRNAs (pre-miRNAs; Lee et al. 2003). The pre-miRNA is then transported to the cytoplasm, where it is subsequently processed by RNase III Dicer into a mature miRNA of approximately 21 nucleotides (Hutvagner et al. 2001). The mature miRNA is then incorporated into the RNA-induced silencing complex (RISC), where mRNA target interaction takes place (Hammond et al. 2000). The canonical model of miRNA-mRNA interaction occurs by perfect or partial pairing at the 5'-end of the miRNA to a complementary site of the 3' UTR of the target. A sequence of 6–8 nucleotides at the 5' end of the miRNA, called the seed region, guides the RISC complex to targeted mRNAs. Repression of mRNAs may then occur by inhibition of translation or by degradation of the transcript, ultimately reducing protein abundance of targeted genes (Melo and Melo 2014).

A key challenge in miRNA research to date involves identifying the target genes for each miRNA. The seed is a dominant motif in miRNAs and is, therefore, used in prediction algorithms to identify potential targets. The algorithms are centred on finding complementary sequences in the 3' UTR of mRNAs. Evolutionary conservation of the complementary sequence is also taken into consideration, and whether there is a supplementary pairing site in the 3' part of the miRNA (for review, see Bartel 2009). However, at present the prediction algorithms have been only partially accurate in identifying true target sites, yielding both false positive and false negative predictions. When comparing results from silencing and over-expression experiments, only a small percentage of mRNA targets were found to be affected by both (Nicolas et al. 2008). Of these, approximately half had a sequence in the 3'-UTR matching the seed, but none was found by prediction programs (Nicolas et al. 2008). Since miRNAs exert their function both at the level of mRNA abundance and at protein abundance, transcriptomic analysis will miss targets that are regulated only at the protein level. To further add to the complexity of miRNA regulation, one gene may be targeted by several different miRNAs. Additionally, the same miRNA may have several target sites on the same gene (Bartel 2009). One miRNA may even have opposing effects on a target gene in different tissues (Lu et al. 2010; Chuang et al. 2015).

Role of miRNAs in the Regulation of Skeletal Muscle Development

Skeletal Muscle Development and Regeneration

Skeletal muscle has been shown to express several RNA species (Gallagher et al. 2010), and dysregulation of skeletal muscle miRNAs has been implicated in a number of different disease states (Williams et al. 2009a; Massart et al. 2016). Skeletal muscle has a large adaptive potential in response to contractile activity. This plasticity is necessary to modify contractile features and adapt metabolic capacity to new requirements following endurance and/or resistance exercise. Skeletal muscle also has a high regenerative capacity in response to injury or damage. Critical to this plasticity and the regenerative potential of skeletal muscle are myogenic progenitor cells, termed satellite cells (Dumont et al. 2015). In adults, satellite cells are quiescent but they can, in response to injury or increased contractile activity, re-enter the cell cycle and proliferate and thereafter differentiate, fuse, and regenerate myofibres.

Skeletal muscle development has been studied extensively in vitro through isolation, growth and differentiation of satellite cells and in vivo during embryogenesis (see Fig. 1). Molecular regulation of cell determination to the myogenic lineage and proliferation of these cells involves the paired box transcription factors PAX3 and PAX7 (Braun and Gautel 2011). Pax3 loss-of-function during embryogenesis in mice results in the absence of musculature in the trunk region due to reduced migration of satellite cells (Bober et al. 1994; Tremblay et al. 1998). While Pax7 deletion in animals has little effect on embryogenic muscle formation (Oustanina et al. 2004), it is essential for satellite cell formation and adult myogenesis (Sambasivan et al. 2011). When activated, satellite cells can migrate and re-enter the cell cycle to start proliferation. The processes of satellite cell commitment and differentiation into multinucleated myotubes are controlled by a group of basic helix-loop-helix transcription factors known as myogenic regulatory factors (MRFs). The MRFs consist of four members: myogenic factor 5 (MYF5), myogenic differentiation 1 (MYOD1), myogenin (MYOG), and myogenic regulatory factor 4 (MRF4). These transcription factors promote terminal differentiation by regulating the expression of several myogenic genes (Braun and Gautel 2011). Satellite cells committed to the myogenic program and myogenesis are termed myoblasts, which typically express PAX7 and early MRFs such as MYOD and MYF5. Expression of these early MRFs is crucial for myoblast maturation because a combined Myod and Myf5 loss-of-function results in the absence of skeletal muscle formation during embryogenesis (Rudnicki et al. 1993). MYF5 and MYOD are considered determination factors required for establishment of myogenic identity since they are upstream transcriptional regulators of late MRFs, MYOG and MRF4 (Braun and Gautel 2011). Myoblasts will leave the cell cycle for terminal differentiation by lowering PAX7 and MYF5 expression while inducing the late MRFs. The late MRFs are important for terminal differentiation, and lack of, for example, Myog in mice leads to postnatal lethality due to muscle deficiency (Hasty et al. 1993).

miRNA Regulation of Myogenesis In vitro and In vivo

miRNAs are important regulators of cell proliferation and differentiation, processes that are critical to proper tissue development and maintenance. The relative expression of miRNAs is tissue dependent, with several miRNAs showing enrichment in skeletal muscle (and heart muscle). These muscle-enriched miRNAs are termed

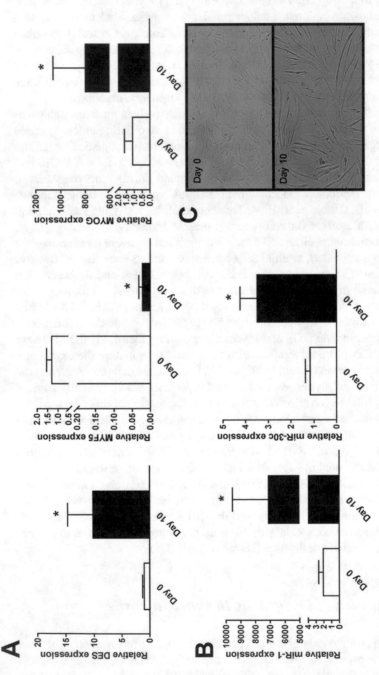

Fig. 1 mRNA and miRNA expression during human skeletal muscle cell differentiation in vitro. Human skeletal muscle cells were cultured until approximately 80% confluence (Day 0; white bars) and induced to differentiate for 10 days (Day 10; black bars). RNA was collected and mRNA and miRNA expression was assessed by RT qPCR. (a) Expression of the myogenic markers desmin (DES), myogenic factor 5 (MYF5) and myogenin (MYOG) before inducing myoblasts to differentiate and following differentiation into myotubes. (b) Expression of a muscle-enriched (miR-1) and a non-muscle-enriched (miR-30c) miRNA before and after differentiation. (c) Representative microscope bright-field pictures of cells prior to inducing differentiation (top) and following myotube formation after differentiation (bottom). All data represent average ± SEM, *p < 0.05 [paired student's t-test (normal distribution of data) or Wilcoxon matched-pairs singed rank test (non-normal distribution of data)]

"myomiRs" (Sempere et al. 2004). Some members of the myomiRs are organized in bicistronic clusters with genomic colocalisation of miR-1-1/miR-133a-2, miR-1-2/miR-133a-1 and miR-133b/206. Thus, these miRNAs share similar expression patterns and are induced during skeletal muscle cell differentiation by upstream transcriptional regulation of different MRF members, including MYOD and MYOG (Rao et al. 2006; Sweetman et al. 2008). Besides sharing similar regulation of expression, they also share similar sequences. For example, miR-133a-1/2 (identical sequences) and miR-133b differ by only one single nucleotide outside of the seed region, and miR-1-1/2 (identical sequences) and miR-206 differ in four nucleotides at the 3' end but share identical seed sequences in humans. Thus, miR-1 and miR-206, and miR-133a and miR-133b, respectively, regulate a set of similar, but not identical, target genes.

The aforementioned myomiRs are all potent regulators of satellite cell differentiation and proliferation. miR-1 and miR-206 are induced upon satellite cell commitment and differentiation, and increased expression promotes differentiation of these cells (Fig. 1; Chen et al. 2006; Kim et al. 2006). miR-1 and miR-206 induce differentiation by targeting several repressors of skeletal muscle cell differentiation, including histone deacetylase 4 (Hdac4); Chen et al. 2006; Williams et al. 2009b), Pax3 (Goljanek-Whysall et al. 2011) and Pax7 (Chen et al. 2010). The effects of miR-133a/b on myogenesis are still debated. It is clear that miR-133, like several other myomiRs, is induced during skeletal muscle differentiation (Chen et al. 2006; Kim et al. 2006), whereas different effects of miR-133 on the myogenic process have been reported. Initial observations have indicated that miR-133 promotes the proliferative state of myoblasts by repressing Serum Response Factor (Srf; Chen et al. 2006). More recent evidence suggests that miR-133 instead functions by inhibiting myoblast proliferation to promote muscle cell differentiation (Zhang et al. 2012; Feng et al. 2013). These effects of miR-133 are due to targeting of pro-proliferative target genes. Such targets include SP1 transcription factor (Sp1), an upstream regulator of Cyclin D1 expression, and Fibroblast Growth Factor Receptor 1 (Fgfr1) and Protein Phosphatase 2 Catalytic Subunit Alpha (Pp2ac), which are important for regulation of ERK1/2 phosphorylation status (Zhang et al. 2012; Feng et al. 2013). The differences in results noted could indicate that miR-133 can influence both proliferation and differentiation in a context-dependent manner.

While the effects of miR-1 and miR-206 on skeletal muscle cell differentiation in vitro are clear, ablation of miR-1-2 or miR-206 in mice did not result in disturbed skeletal muscle development during embryogenesis in vivo (Zhao et al. 2007; Williams et al. 2009b). Nevertheless, genetic deletion of miR-206 negatively affected post-embryonic regeneration of muscle and neuromuscular connections following injury (Williams et al. 2009b; Liu et al. 2012). Furthermore, miR-206 deletion exacerbated the dystrophic phenotype in a mouse model of muscular dystrophy (Liu et al. 2012). Contrary to these results, deletion of the miR-206/miR-133b cluster was found not to be required for proper muscle regeneration (Boettger et al. 2014). These differences, and the absence of a robust phenotype following myomiR loss-of-function during embryogenesis, could be explained by the large redundancy in this group of myomiRs. Not only are there several genomic copies of miR-1 and miR-133a, but they also share similar sequences with miR-206 and miR-133b, respectively. Thus, miR-1 and miR-133a could compensate for the loss of miR-206/133b expression (Boettger et al. 2014). In contrast, *D. melanogaster* has only one genomic copy of miR-1 and, in this context, the absence of miR-206 is coincident with severely deformed musculature in miR-1 mutant larvae (Sokol and Ambros 2005), implicating that the presence of several genomic copies, as found in other species, provides system redundancy. Furthermore, a double knockout of miR-133a-1 and miR-133a-2 in mice resulted in cardiomyopathy and lethal defects in approximately 50% of offspring, whereas mice lacking only miR-133a-1 or miR-133a-2 did not show this phenotype (Liu et al. 2008). The miR-133a double knockout mice that survived until adulthood also showed skeletal muscle defects, including mitochondrial dysfunction and centronuclear myopathy of type II fibres (Liu et al. 2011).

Skeletal muscle-specific Dicer ablation in mice results in reduced muscle-specific miRNA expression and perinatal death, abnormal muscle morphology and reduced skeletal muscle mass (O'Rourke et al. 2007), indicating that proper miRNA maturation is essential for overall muscle function and development. Conditional knockout of Dicer in satellite cells in adult mice results in satellite cells exiting quiescence and entering the cell cycle, leading to severely impaired regeneration following skeletal muscle injury (Cheung et al. 2012). Collectively, evidence points towards a central function of miRNAs, not only for normal embryonic skeletal muscle biogenesis but also for adult muscle function and repair.

Not only is the expression of several myomiRs altered in response to satellite cell expansion and differentiation, but also several non-muscle enriched miRNAs are temporally regulated in expression during muscle cell differentiation (see Fig. 1). Several studies have determined miRNA expression profiles during differentiation in vitro and during myogenesis in vivo (Chen et al. 2011; Cheung et al. 2012; Koning et al. 2012; Dmitriev et al. 2013; Sjögren et al. 2015). We identified 44 miRNAs, including the canonical myomiRs, to be altered during primary human skeletal muscle cell differentiation (Sjögren et al. 2015), comparable to the 60 miRNAs altered in a similar study (Dmitriev et al. 2013). Nevertheless, these miRNAs might not influence either the proliferation or differentiation process but may be involved in other phenotypic changes associated with muscle cell differentiation, such as metabolism, hypertrophy or mitochondrial function. Examples of non-muscle-enriched miRNAs identified to have altered expression and directly affecting proliferation or differentiation of skeletal muscle cells include, for example, miR-26a (Dey et al. 2012), miR-30 (Fig. 1; Guess et al. 2015) and miR-199a-5p (Alexander et al. 2013). Future studies are required to determine the targets and effects on skeletal muscle cell proliferation and differentiation, both in vivo and in vitro, of several of the miRNAs that have altered expression during satellite cell activation and differentiation.

Skeletal Muscle miRNA in Metabolic Disease

Approximately half of the total body mass in healthy individuals consists of skeletal muscle, representing a substantial part of whole-body metabolism (DeFronzo and Tripathy 2009). Skeletal muscle also represents a primary target for insulin-mediated glucose disposal, and skeletal muscle insulin resistance is a characteristic feature in type 2 diabetes and in conditions of impaired glucose metabolism transport activity (Krook et al. 2000; Ryder et al. 2000). Furthermore, skeletal muscle function is crucial for proper posturing and locomotion patterns, and disruption in metabolic or motile functionality may greatly decrease an individual's quality of life. While there is good evidence that miRNAs play a key role in the regulation of muscle growth and differentiation, dysregulation of skeletal muscle miRNA expression in disease states has been less well studied, in particular in human cohorts.

Several miRNAs were found to be downregulated in response to a 3-h euglycaemic-hyperinsulinaemic clamp in human skeletal muscle, including miR-1 and miR-133a (Granjon et al. 2009). Expression profiles of skeletal muscle miR-NAs have been reported in a number of different rodent models of obesity and diabetes, including Goto-Kakizaki (GK) rats, a non-obese spontaneous T2D model (He et al. 2007a; Huang et al. 2009; Herrera et al. 2010), rats rendered diabetic by a combination of high fat diet and a low dose of streptozotocin (Karolina et al. 2011), as well as mice fed a high fat diet (Chen et al. 2012; Mohamed et al. 2014). These different models share skeletal muscle insulin resistance as a key characteristic. When miRNA profiles from patients with type 2 diabetes were compared against these different animal models, eight upregulated miRNAs found in type 2 diabetic patients were also found to be upregulated in at least one of the rodent arrays (for review and analysis, see Massart et al. 2016). Similarly, 16 of the downregulated miRNAs were recapitulated in rodent studies. Interestingly, two thirds of the commonly regulated miRNAs have been identified in mice rendered insulin resistant in response to a high fat diet (Massart et al. 2016). However, different miRNAs showed altered expression depending on the model. For example, miR-99a and miR-100, which were downregulated in skeletal muscle from patients with type 2 diabetes and in mice fed a high fat diet, were upregulated in rats on a high fat diet rendered diabetic with streptozotocin, suggesting that the aetiology of the insulin resistance influenced the miRNA expression signature. As yet, only a few of these miRNAs have been studied in vitro and/or in vivo in relation to metabolic disease, and their targets remain poorly characterized.

Skeletal Muscle miRNAs in Response to Exercise

Skeletal muscle responds rapidly to exercise, and even a single bout of acute exercise is sufficient to induce changes in gene expression. In response to many bouts of acute exercise, i.e., exercise training, skeletal muscle adapts by altering protein production, which impacts the functional as well as the metabolic properties of the exercised muscle. The inter-individual variability in skeletal muscle hypertrophic response to resistance exercise has been attributed to variations in the ability of satellite cell mobilization to proliferate and subsequent fuse with existing muscle fibres (Petrella et al. 2006, 2008). As detailed above, several miRNAs regulate skeletal muscle satellite cell quiescence, activation and differentiation, indicating potential roles for these miRNAs in skeletal muscle hypertrophy.

Identification of pathways and molecular mechanisms regulating skeletal muscle exercise adaptation has been a key focus from a number of different angles; from probing understanding of athletic performance to alterations relevant for metabolic disease. Different modes of exercise training lead to different adaptive responses; for example, strength training leads to more hypertrophic responses whereas aerobic exercise increases endurance. These differences are also mirrored in the different intracellular signalling pathways that are activated (for review, see Egan and Zierath 2013). Several lines of evidence suggest an important role for miRNAs in skeletal muscle development and hypertrophy (for review see Zacharewicz et al. 2013; Kovanda et al. 2014).

Several human studies have reported that short exercise bouts/training duration lead to increased skeletal muscle expression of miR-1 (Nielsen et al. 2010; Russell et al. 2013), whereas longer endurance training protocols lead to miR-1 downregulation (Nielsen et al. 2010; Drummond et al. 2011; Keller et al. 2011). Rodent studies are in general agreement regarding regulation of myomiRs in response to exercise (for review see Zacharewicz et al. 2013). In contrast, although several of the classical myomiRs have been noted to respond to exercise, a clear consensus has yet to emerge regarding which other miRNAs are regulated in response to exercise. These inconsistencies in the literature may be due to species differences as well as differences in the exercise protocols used, but they may even depend on different RNA extraction protocols (for more in depth discussion see Zacharewicz et al. 2013).

miRNA Regulation of Skeletal Muscle Atrophy and During States of Muscle Mass Loss

Skeletal muscle is the largest organ in adult mammals and muscle function is critical to metabolic homeostasis and health across the whole life span. Loss of skeletal muscle mass (atrophy) and function, also referred to as sarcopenia, occurs with aging (Cartee et al. 2016). Muscle loss is also noted in obese individuals, a phenomenon known as sarcopenic obesity, and is associated with lowered skeletal muscle insulin sensitivity. In addition, individuals with cancer, HIV-AIDS, chronic heart failure, chronic obstructive pulmonary disease, renal failure, rheumatoid arthritis, and osteoarthritis can all experience a dramatic loss of muscle mass (Wolfe 2006). Thus understanding the regulation of skeletal muscle mass and function is of clinical relevance.

Three members of the myomiR family, miR-208a, miR-208b and miR-499, are encoded and expressed from sequences embedded within heart- and skeletal muscle-enriched myosin genes, MYH6, MYH7 and MYH7B, respectively (van Rooij et al. 2009). miR-208a is exclusively expressed in heart muscle, whereas miR-208b and miR-499 are expressed both in heart muscle and in type I (oxidative) skeletal muscle fibres. Loss of function of both miR-208b and miR-499 in mice results in loss of type I fibres and is associated with increased expression of miR-208b and miR-499 pro-atrophic target genes, including purine rich element binding protein beta (Purb) and SRY-box containing gene 6 (Sox6; van Rooij et al. 2009). Furthermore, four weeks of hind limb suspension, resulting in severe skeletal muscle atrophy, reduces expression of miR-208b and miR-499 in rat skeletal muscle (McCarthy et al. 2009). In humans with skeletal muscle loss due to spinal cord injury, expression of miR-208b and miR-499-5p is reduced and inversely related to expression of myostatin, a critical regulator of skeletal muscle mass (Boon et al. 2015). These miRNAs also participate in a transcriptional network together with estrogen-related receptors (ERRs) and members of the peroxisome proliferator activated receptor (PPAR) family to coordinate the regulation of skeletal muscle energy metabolism and fibre type specification (Gan et al. 2013).

Muscular dystrophy is characterized by muscle atrophy and weakness. A large microarray-based study found expression of 185 miRNAs to be altered in skeletal muscle in at least one of 10 common muscular disorders, including Duchenne muscular dystrophy (DMD; Eisenberg et al. 2007). Several miRNAs have been noted to be dysregulated both in human Duchenne muscular dystrophy and in a mouse model of the disease (Greco et al. 2009). Examples of dysregulated miRNAs include miR-206, which was upregulated in states of muscular dystrophy (McCarthy et al. 2007; Greco et al. 2009), potentially due to constant regenerative processes in dystrophic skeletal muscle. However, as mentioned above, mice lacking miR-206 have a muscle dystrophic phenotype (Liu et al. 2012), underscoring the complexity of miRNA regulation. In the case of muscular dystrophy, a number of miRNAs has been proposed to have possible therapeutic potential. For example, overexpression of miR-486, another muscle-enriched miRNA with decreased expression in muscle dystrophy (Eisenberg et al. 2007), improved muscle function in a mouse model of muscle dystrophy (Alexander et al. 2014). Another example is miR-431, where transgenic miR-431 mice with muscular dystrophy have improved skeletal muscle fatigability and force generation, potentially due to improved muscle regeneration and enhanced muscle cell differentiation capacity in vitro (Wu et al. 2015).

miRNAs are also potent regulators of signalling pathways known to regulate muscle atrophy. Two critical regulators of skeletal muscle atrophy are F-box Protein 32 [FBXO32; also known as Muscle atrophy F-box (MAFbx)] and Tripartite Motif Containing 63 [TRIM63; also known as Muscle RING finger 1 (MuRF1)], which regulate protein degradation through regulation of ubiquitination. The family of Forkhead Box O (FOXO) transcription factors, especially FOXO1 and FOXO3, are strong upstream regulators of both these genes during skeletal muscle atrophy (Glass 2010). FOXO1 activity was reduced following miR-486 overexpression in skeletal muscle cells in vitro, both through decreased FOXO1 expression and through increased FOXO1 phosphorylation (inhibitory) through direct miR-486-

targeting of Phosphatase and Tensin Homolog (PTEN), a negative regulator of FOXO1-upstream kinase AKT (Xu et al. 2012). miR-486 overexpression also reduced induction of FOXO1 targets MAFbx and MuRF-1 protein expression in primary mouse muscle cells following treatment with dexamethasone, a potent inducer of muscle atrophy (Xu et al. 2012). In addition, overexpression of miR-486 protected against skeletal muscle loss in a mouse model of chronic kidney disease (Xu et al. 2012). Furthermore, miR-486 inhibition in vitro slightly reduced myotube diameter, and inhibition in vivo reduced the cross-sectional area of muscle fibres, confirming the effects of miR-486 on regulation of skeletal muscle mass (Hitachi et al. 2014). MAFbx and MuRF1 are also directly under miRNA-dependent regulation by two different miRNAs, miR-23a and miR-23b (Wada et al. 2011). miR-23a overexpression either in vitro or with a transgene in mouse skeletal muscle protected against dexamethasone-induced muscle atrophy (Wada et al. 2011). Cellular miR-23a is decreased in dexamethasone-induced skeletal muscle atrophy, potentially through a mechanism including enhanced exosomal release of miR-23a (Hudson et al. 2014).

miRNA expression has also been assessed following age or sarcopenia-induced skeletal muscle loss (Drummond et al. 2011; Rivas et al. 2014; Zacharewicz et al. 2014). Nevertheless, the overlap of miRNA signatures is small between these studies, potentially due to the small number of biological replicates in each study or due to different platforms to assess miRNA expression. Further studies will be needed to determine the impact of miRNA expression and regulation of target genes in human sarcopenia and muscle loss with ageing.

Conclusions

miRNAs are critical regulators of skeletal muscle function and play important roles in maintaining muscle function and regulating adaptation to different situations, including muscle use and disuse, as well as in different disease states. While the role of some of the classical myomiRs is increasingly appreciated and well understood, the challenge for the field lies in understanding not only the precise regulation of different miRNA species but also in dissecting and understanding the precise targets regulated by each miRNA or combination of miRNAs. Unravelling these molecular signatures could facilitate targeted and tissue-specific miRNA interventions in different disease states affecting skeletal muscle function and metabolism.

References

Alexander MS, Kawahara G, Motohashi N, Casar JC, Eisenberg I, Myers JA, Gasperini MJ, Estrella EA, Kho AT, Mitsuhashi S, Shapiro F, Kang PB, Kunkel LM (2013) MicroRNA-199a is induced in dystrophic muscle and affects WNT signaling, cell proliferation, and myogenic differentiation. Cell Death Differ 20:1194–1208

Alexander MS, Casar JC, Motohashi N, Vieira NM, Eisenberg I, Marshall JL, Gasperini MJ, Lek A, Myers JA, Estrella EA, Kang PB, Shapiro F, Rahimov F, Kawahara G, Widrick JJ, Kunkel LM (2014) MicroRNA-486-dependent modulation of DOCK3/PTEN/AKT signaling pathways improves muscular dystrophy-associated symptoms. J Clin Invest 124:2651–2667

Bartel DP (2009) MicroRNAs: target recognition and regulatory functions. Cell 136:215–233

Bober E, Franz T, Arnold HH, Gruss P, Tremblay P (1994) Pax-3 is required for the development of limb muscles: a possible role for the migration of dermomyotomal muscle progenitor cells. Development 120:603–612

Boettger T, Wust S, Nolte H, Braun T (2014) The miR-206/133b cluster is dispensable for development, survival and regeneration of skeletal muscle. Skelet Muscle 4:23

Boon H, Sjögren RJ, Massart J, Egan B, Kostovski E, Iversen PO, Hjeltnes N, Chibalin AV, Widegren U, Zierath JR (2015) MicroRNA-208b progressively declines after spinal cord injury in humans and is inversely related to myostatin expression. Physiol Rep 3. pii: e12622

Braun T, Gautel M (2011) Transcriptional mechanisms regulating skeletal muscle differentiation, growth and homeostasis. Nat Rev Mol Cell Biol 12:349–361

Cartee GD, Hepple RT, Bamman MM, Zierath JR (2016) Exercise promotes healthy aging of skeletal muscle. Cell Metab 23:1034–1047

Chen JF, Mandel EM, Thomson JM, Wu Q, Callis TE, Hammond SM, Conlon FL, Wang DZ (2006) The role of microRNA-1 and microRNA-133 in skeletal muscle proliferation and differentiation. Nat Genet 38:228–233

Chen JF, Tao Y, Li J, Deng Z, Yan Z, Xiao X, Wang DZ (2010) microRNA-1 and microRNA-206 regulate skeletal muscle satellite cell proliferation and differentiation by repressing Pax7. J Cell Biol 190:867–879

Chen Y, Gelfond J, McManus LM, Shireman PK (2011) Temporal microRNA expression during in vitro myogenic progenitor cell proliferation and differentiation: regulation of proliferation by miR-682. Physiol Genomics 43:621–630

Chen GQ, Lian WJ, Wang GM, Wang S, Yang YQ, Zhao ZW (2012) Altered microRNA expression in skeletal muscle results from high-fat diet-induced insulin resistance in mice. Mol Med Rep 5:1362–1368

Cheung TH, Quach NL, Charville GW, Liu L, Park L, Edalati A, Yoo B, Hoang P, Rando TA (2012) Maintenance of muscle stem-cell quiescence by microRNA-489. Nature 482:524–528

Chuang TY, Wu HL, Chen CC, Gamboa GM, Layman LC, Diamond MP, Azziz R, Chen YH (2015) MicroRNA-223 expression is upregulated in insulin resistant human adipose tissue. J Diabet Res 2015:943659

DeFronzo RA, Tripathy D (2009) Skeletal muscle insulin resistance is the primary defect in type 2 diabetes. Diabetes Care 32(Suppl 2):S157–S163

Dey BK, Gagan J, Yan Z, Dutta A (2012) miR-26a is required for skeletal muscle differentiation and regeneration in mice. Genes Dev 26:2180–2191

Dmitriev P, Barat A, Polesskaya A, O'Connell MJ, Robert T, Dessen P, Walsh TA, Lazar V, Turki A, Carnac G, Laoudj-Chenivesse D, Lipinski M, Vassetzky YS (2013) Simultaneous miRNA and mRNA transcriptome profiling of human myoblasts reveals a novel set of myogenic differentiation-associated miRNAs and their target genes. BMC Genomics 14:265

Drummond MJ, McCarthy JJ, Sinha M, Spratt DM, Volpi E, Esser KA, Rasmussen BB (2011) Aging and microRNA expression in human skeletal muscle: a microarray and bioinformatics analysis. Physiol Genomics 43:595–603

Dumont NA, Bentzinger CF, Sincennes MC, Rudnicki MA (2015) Satellite cells and skeletal muscle regeneration. Compr Physiol 5:1027–1059

Egan B, Zierath JR (2013) Exercise metabolism and the molecular regulation of skeletal muscle adaptation. Cell Metab 17:162–184

Eisenberg I, Eran A, Nishino I, Moggio M, Lamperti C, Amato AA, Lidov HG, Kang PB, North KN, Mitrani-Rosenbaum S, Flanigan KM, Neely LA, Whitney D, Beggs AH, Kohane IS, Kunkel LM (2007) Distinctive patterns of microRNA expression in primary muscular disorders. Proc Natl Acad Sci USA 104:17016–17021

Feng Y, Niu LL, Wei W, Zhang WY, Li XY, Cao JH, Zhao SH (2013) A feedback circuit between miR-133 and the ERK1/2 pathway involving an exquisite mechanism for regulating myoblast proliferation and differentiation. Cell Death Dis 4:e934

Gallagher IJ, Scheele C, Keller P, Nielsen AR, Remenyi J, Fischer CP, Roder K, Babraj J, Wahlestedt C, Hutvagner G, Pedersen BK, Timmons JA (2010) Integration of microRNA changes in vivo identifies novel molecular features of muscle insulin resistance in type 2 diabetes. Genome Med 2:9

Gan Z, Rumsey J, Hazen BC, Lai L, Leone TC, Vega RB, Xie H, Conley KE, Auwerx J, Smith SR, Olson EN, Kralli A, Kelly DP (2013) Nuclear receptor/microRNA circuitry links muscle fiber type to energy metabolism. J Clin Invest 123:2564–2575

Glass DJ (2010) Signaling pathways perturbing muscle mass. Curr Opin Clin Nutr Metab Care 13:225–229

Goljanek-Whysall K, Sweetman D, Abu-Elmagd M, Chapnik E, Dalmay T, Hornstein E, Munsterberg A (2011) MicroRNA regulation of the paired-box transcription factor Pax3 confers robustness to developmental timing of myogenesis. Proc Natl Acad Sci USA 108:11936–11941

Granjon A, Gustin M-P, Rieusset J, Lefai E, Meugnier E, Güller I, Cerutti C, Paultre C, Disse E, Rabasa-Lhoret R, Laville M, Vidal H, Rome S (2009) The microRNA signature in response to insulin reveals its implication in the transcriptional action of insulin in human skeletal muscle and the role of a sterol regulatory element–binding protein-1c/myocyte enhancer factor 2C pathway. Diabetes 58:2555–2564

Greco S, De Simone M, Colussi C, Zaccagnini G, Fasanaro P, Pescatori M, Cardani R, Perbellini R, Isaia E, Sale P, Meola G, Capogrossi MC, Gaetano C, Martelli F (2009) Common micro-RNA signature in skeletal muscle damage and regeneration induced by Duchenne muscular dystrophy and acute ischemia. FASEB J 23:3335–3346

Guess MG, Barthel KK, Harrison BC, Leinwand LA (2015) miR-30 family microRNAs regulate myogenic differentiation and provide negative feedback on the microRNA pathway. PLoS One 10:e0118229

Hammond SM, Bernstein E, Beach D, Hannon GJ (2000) An RNA-directed nuclease mediates post-transcriptional gene silencing in Drosophila cells. Nature 404:293–296

Hasty P, Bradley A, Morris JH, Edmondson DG, Venuti JM, Olson EN, Klein WH (1993) Muscle deficiency and neonatal death in mice with a targeted mutation in the myogenin gene. Nature 364:501–506

He A, Zhu L, Gupta N, Chang Y, Fang F (2007a) Overexpression of micro ribonucleic acid 29, highly up-regulated in diabetic rats, leads to insulin resistance in 3T3-L1 adipocytes. Mol Endocrinol 21:2785–2794

He L, He X, Lowe SW, Hannon GJ (2007b) microRNAs join the p53 network—another piece in the tumour-suppression puzzle. Nat Rev Cancer 7:819–822

Herrera BM, Lockstone HE, Taylor JM, Ria M, Barrett A, Collins S, Kaisaki P, Argoud K, Fernandez C, Travers ME, Grew JP, Randall JC, Gloyn AL, Gauguier D, McCarthy MI, Lindgren CM (2010) Global microRNA expression profiles in insulin target tissues in a spontaneous rat model of type 2 diabetes. Diabetologia 53:1099–1109

Hitachi K, Nakatani M, Tsuchida K (2014) Myostatin signaling regulates Akt activity via the regulation of miR-486 expression. Intl J. Biochem Cell Biol 47:93–103

Huang B, Qin W, Zhao B, Shi Y, Yao C, Li J, Xiao H, Jin Y (2009) MicroRNA expression profiling in diabetic GK rat model. Acta Biochim Biophys Sin 41:472–477

Hudson MB, Woodworth-Hobbs ME, Zheng B, Rahnert JA, Blount MA, Gooch JL, Searles CD, Price SR (2014) miR-23a is decreased during muscle atrophy by a mechanism that includes calcineurin signaling and exosome-mediated export. Am J Physiol Cell Physiol 306:C551–C558

Hutvagner G, McLachlan J, Pasquinelli AE, Balint E, Tuschl T, Zamore PD (2001) A cellular function for the RNA-interference enzyme Dicer in the maturation of the let-7 small temporal RNA. Science 293:834–838

Karolina DS, Armugam A, Tavintharan S, Wong MT, Lim SC, Sum CF, Jeyaseelan K (2011) MicroRNA 144 impairs insulin signaling by inhibiting the expression of insulin receptor substrate 1 in type 2 diabetes mellitus. PLoS One 6:e22839

Keller P, Vollaard NBJ, Gustafsson T, Gallagher IJ, Sundberg CJ, Rankinen T, Britton SL, Bouchard C, Koch LG, Timmons JA (2011) A transcriptional map of the impact of endurance exercise training on skeletal muscle phenotype. J Appl Physiol 110:46–59

Kim HK, Lee YS, Sivaprasad U, Malhotra A, Dutta A (2006) Muscle-specific microRNA miR-206 promotes muscle differentiation. J Cell Biol 174:677–687

Koning M, Werker PM, van Luyn MJ, Krenning G, Harmsen MC (2012) A global downregulation of microRNAs occurs in human quiescent satellite cells during myogenesis. Differentiation 84:314–321

Kovanda A, Režen T, Rogelj B (2014) MicroRNA in skeletal muscle development, growth, atrophy, and disease. Wiley Interdiscip Rev RNA 5:509–525

Krook A, Bjornholm M, Galuska D, Jiang XJ, Fahlman R, Myers MG Jr, Wallberg-Henriksson H, Zierath JR (2000) Characterization of signal transduction and glucose transport in skeletal muscle from type 2 diabetic patients. Diabetes 49:284–292

Lee RC, Feinbaum RL, Ambros V (1993) The C. elegans heterochronic gene lin-4 encodes small RNAs with antisense complementarity to lin-14. Cell 75:843–854

Lee Y, Ahn C, Han J, Choi H, Kim J, Yim J, Lee J, Provost P, Radmark O, Kim S, Kim VN (2003) The nuclear RNase III Drosha initiates microRNA processing. Nature 425:415–419

Liu N, Bezprozvannaya S, Williams AH, Qi X, Richardson JA, Bassel-Duby R, Olson EN (2008) microRNA-133a regulates cardiomyocyte proliferation and suppresses smooth muscle gene expression in the heart. Genes Dev 22:3242–3254

Liu N, Bezprozvannaya S, Shelton JM, Frisard MI, Hulver MW, McMillan RP, Wu Y, Voelker KA, Grange RW, Richardson JA, Bassel-Duby R, Olson EN (2011) Mice lacking microRNA 133a develop dynamin 2-dependent centronuclear myopathy. J Clin Invest 121:3258–3268

Liu N, Williams AH, Maxeiner JM, Bezprozvannaya S, Shelton JM, Richardson JA, Bassel-Duby R, Olson EN (2012) microRNA-206 promotes skeletal muscle regeneration and delays progression of Duchenne muscular dystrophy in mice. J Clin Invest 122:2054–2065

Lu H, Buchan RJ, Cook SA (2010) MicroRNA-223 regulates Glut4 expression and cardiomyocyte glucose metabolism. Cardiovasc Res 86:410–420

Massart J, Katayama M, Krook A (2016) microManaging glucose and lipid metabolism in skeletal muscle: role of microRNAs. Biochim Biophys Acta 1861:2130–2138

McCarthy JJ, Esser KA, Andrade FH (2007) MicroRNA-206 is overexpressed in the diaphragm but not the hindlimb muscle of mdx mouse. Am J Physiol Cell Physiol 293:C451–C457

McCarthy JJ, Esser KA, Peterson CA, Dupont-Versteegden EE (2009) Evidence of MyomiR network regulation of beta-myosin heavy chain gene expression during skeletal muscle atrophy. Physiol Genomics 39:219–226

Melo CA, Melo SA (2014) Biogenesis and physiology of microRNAs. In: Fabbri M (ed) Noncoding RNAs and cancer. Springer, New York, pp 5–24

Mohamed JS, Hajira A, Pardo PS, Boriek AM (2014) MicroRNA-149 inhibits PARP-2 and promotes mitochondrial biogenesis via SIRT-1/PGC-1α network in skeletal muscle. Diabetes 63:1546–1559

Nicolas FE, Pais H, Schwach F, Lindow M, Kauppinen S, Moulton V, Dalmay T (2008) Experimental identification of microRNA-140 targets by silencing and overexpressing miR-140. RNA 14:2513 2520

Nielsen S, Scheele C, Yfanti C, Åkerström T, Nielsen AR, Pedersen BK, Laye M (2010) Muscle specific microRNAs are regulated by endurance exercise in human skeletal muscle. J Physiol 588:4029–4037

O'Rourke JR, Georges SA, Seay HR, Tapscott SJ, McManus MT, Goldhamer DJ, Swanson MS, Harfe BD (2007) Essential role for Dicer during skeletal muscle development. Dev Biol 311:359–368

Oustanina S, Hause G, Braun T (2004) Pax7 directs postnatal renewal and propagation of myogenic satellite cells but not their specification. EMBO J 23:3430–3439

Petrella JK, Kim JS, Cross JM, Kosek DJ, Bamman MM (2006) Efficacy of myonuclear addition may explain differential myofiber growth among resistance-trained young and older men and women. Am J Physiol Endocrinol Metab 291:E937–E946

Petrella JK, Kim JS, Mayhew DL, Cross JM, Bamman MM (2008) Potent myofiber hypertrophy during resistance training in humans is associated with satellite cell-mediated myonuclear addition: a cluster analysis. J Appl Physiol (1985) 104:1736–1742

Rao PK, Kumar RM, Farkhondeh M, Baskerville S, Lodish HF (2006) Myogenic factors that regulate expression of muscle-specific microRNAs. Proc Natl Acad Sci USA 103:8721–8726

Reinhart BJ, Slack FJ, Basson M, Pasquinelli AE, Bettinger JC, Rougvie AE, Horvitz HR, Ruvkun G (2000) The 21-nucleotide let-7 RNA regulates developmental timing in Caenorhabditis elegans. Nature 403:901–906

Rivas DA, Lessard SJ, Rice NP, Lustgarten MS, So K, Goodyear LJ, Parnell LD, Fielding RA (2014) Diminished skeletal muscle microRNA expression with aging is associated with attenuated muscle plasticity and inhibition of IGF-1 signaling. FASEB J 28:4133–4147

Rudnicki MA, Schnegelsberg PN, Stead RH, Braun T, Arnold HH, Jaenisch R (1993) MyoD or Myf-5 is required for the formation of skeletal muscle. Cell 75:1351–1359

Russell AP, Lamon S, Boon H, Wada S, Güller I, Brown EL, Chibalin AV, Zierath JR, Snow RJ, Stepto N, Wadley GD, Akimoto T (2013) Regulation of miRNAs in human skeletal muscle following acute endurance exercise and short-term endurance training. J Physiol 591:4637–4653

Ryder JW, Yang J, Galuska D, Rincon J, Bjornholm M, Krook A, Lund S, Pedersen O, Wallberg-Henriksson H, Zierath JR, Holman GD (2000) Use of a novel impermeable biotinylated photolabeling reagent to assess insulin- and hypoxia-stimulated cell surface GLUT4 content in skeletal muscle from type 2 diabetic patients. Diabetes 49:647–654

Sambasivan R, Yao R, Kissenpfennig A, Van Wittenberghe L, Paldi A, Gayraud-Morel B, Guenou H, Malissen B, Tajbakhsh S, Galy A (2011) Pax7-expressing satellite cells are indispensable for adult skeletal muscle regeneration. Development 138:3647–3656

Sempere LF, Freemantle S, Pitha-Rowe I, Moss E, Dmitrovsky E, Ambros V (2004) Expression profiling of mammalian microRNAs uncovers a subset of brain-expressed microRNAs with possible roles in murine and human neuronal differentiation. Genome Biol 5:R13

Sjögren RJ, Egan B, Katayama M, Zierath JR, Krook A (2015) Temporal analysis of reciprocal miRNA-mRNA expression patterns predicts regulatory networks during differentiation in human skeletal muscle cells. Physiol Genomics 47:45–57

Sokol NS, Ambros V (2005) Mesodermally expressed Drosophila microRNA-1 is regulated by twist and is required in muscles during larval growth. Genes Dev 19:2343–2354

Sweetman D, Goljanek K, Rathjen T, Oustanina S, Braun T, Dalmay T, Munsterberg A (2008) Specific requirements of MRFs for the expression of muscle specific microRNAs, miR-1, miR-206 and miR-133. Dev Biol 321:491–499

Tremblay P, Dietrich S, Mericskay M, Schubert FR, Li Z, Paulin D (1998) A crucial role for Pax3 in the development of the hypaxial musculature and the long-range migration of muscle precursors. Dev Biol 203:49–61

van Rooij E, Quiat D, Johnson BA, Sutherland LB, Qi X, Richardson JA, Kelm RJ Jr, Olson EN (2009) A family of microRNAs encoded by myosin genes governs myosin expression and muscle performance. Dev Cell 17:662–673

Wada S, Kato Y, Okutsu M, Miyaki S, Suzuki K, Yan Z, Schiaffino S, Asahara H, Ushida T, Akimoto T (2011) Translational suppression of atrophic regulators by microRNA-23a integrates resistance to skeletal muscle atrophy. J Biol Chem 286:38456–38465

Wightman B, Ha I, Ruvkun G (1993) Posttranscriptional regulation of the heterochronic gene lin-14 by lin-4 mediates temporal pattern formation in C. elegans. Cell 75:855–862

Williams AH, Liu N, van Rooij E, Olson EN (2009a) MicroRNA control of muscle development and disease. Curr Opin Cell Biol 21:461–469

Williams AH, Valdez G, Moresi V, Qi X, McAnally J, Elliott JL, Bassel-Duby R, Sanes JR, Olson EN (2009b) MicroRNA-206 delays ALS progression and promotes regeneration of neuromuscular synapses in mice. Science 326:1549–1554

Wolfe RR (2006) The underappreciated role of muscle in health and disease. Am J Clin Nutr 84:475–482

Wu R, Li H, Zhai L, Zou X, Meng J, Zhong R, Li C, Wang H, Zhang Y, Zhu D (2015) MicroRNA-431 accelerates muscle regeneration and ameliorates muscular dystrophy by targeting Pax7 in mice. Nat Commun 6:7713

Xu J, Li R, Workeneh B, Dong Y, Wang X, Hu Z (2012) Transcription factor FoxO1, the dominant mediator of muscle wasting in chronic kidney disease, is inhibited by microRNA-486. Kidney Int 82:401–411

Zacharewicz E, Lamon S, Russell A (2013) MicroRNAs in skeletal muscle and their regulation with exercise, ageing, and disease. Front Physiol 4:266

Zacharewicz E, Della Gatta P, Reynolds J, Garnham A, Crowley T, Russell AP, Lamon S (2014) Identification of microRNAs linked to regulators of muscle protein synthesis and regeneration in young and old skeletal muscle. PLoS One 9:e114009

Zhang D, Li X, Chen C, Li Y, Zhao L, Jing Y, Liu W, Wang X, Zhang Y, Xia H, Chang Y, Gao X, Yan J, Ying H (2012) Attenuation of p38-mediated miR-1/133 expression facilitates myoblast proliferation during the early stage of muscle regeneration. PLoS One 7:e41478

Zhao Y, Ransom JF, Li A, Vedantham V, von Drehle M, Muth AN, Tsuchihashi T, McManus MT, Schwartz RJ, Srivastava D (2007) Dysregulation of cardiogenesis, cardiac conduction, and cell cycle in mice lacking miRNA-1-2. Cell 129:303–317

Tryptophan-Kynurenine Metabolites in Exercise and Mental Health

Paula Valente-Silva and Jorge Lira Ruas

Abstract In our efforts to identify molecular mediators of the benefits of exercise to human health, we have uncovered a biochemical pathway in skeletal muscle that positively impacts mental health. This mechanism is activated by endurance training and controlled by the transcriptional coactivator PGC-1α1, which induces transcription of several kynurenine aminotransferase (KAT) genes in muscle. KAT enzymes catabolize the neuroinflammatory tryptophan metabolite kynurenine, which can accumulate in the brain and lead to alterations associated with stress-induced depression (among other psychiatric diseases). Here, we discuss our findings in the context of what is known about the kynurenine pathway of tryptophan degradation and how its many metabolites can directly affect the brain. These findings provide a mechanism for how physical exercise can improve mental health and offers potential therapeutic targets for future antidepressant medications.

Introduction

The many benefits of physical exercise to human health are widely recognized. Depending on their type, intensity, duration, and frequency, different exercise modalities can be used to improve diverse physiological parameters (Hawley et al. 2014). These include cardiovascular fitness, strength, energy metabolism, and resistance to fatigue, among others. Importantly, exercise training can be used as a prophylactic or therapeutic intervention for a variety of pathologies ranging from obesity and diabetes to cancer and mental health disorders (Cooper et al. 2017; Hawley 2004). Indeed, maintaining an active lifestyle continues to be the best way to promote healthy longevity. However, the molecular mechanisms that allow the human body to adapt to exercise challenges are still poorly understood. This is true

P. Valente-Silva • J. L. Ruas (✉)
Department of Physiology and Pharmacology, Molecular and Cellular Exercise Physiology,
Karolinska Institutet, Stockholm, Sweden
e-mail: jorge.ruas@ki.se

© The Author(s) 2017
B. Spiegelman (ed.), *Hormones, Metabolism and the Benefits of Exercise*,
Research and Perspectives in Endocrine Interactions,
https://doi.org/10.1007/978-3-319-72790-5_7

83

for individual tissues and organs but even more so for the network of inter-organ communication events that coordinates whole-body adaptation to the multitude of stimuli that exercise training entails. Skeletal muscle plays a central role in this process and has been the most studied tissue in this context. From this work, we have learned valuable information about key players in the regulation of muscle function, such as the peroxisome proliferator-activated receptor (PPAR)-γ coactivator-1α (PGC-1α) proteins (Correia et al. 2015). This still expanding family of transcriptional coactivators is composed of several splicing variants with different biological activities and discrete regulation, important for the many effects of physical exercise (Martínez-Redondo et al. 2015). By understanding these mechanisms, we have also started to elucidate how myokines (muscle-derived factors with local and/or distal effects) communicate to the rest of the body the changes in skeletal muscle elicited by exercise (Giudice and Taylor 2017). For example, exercise training can reduce the levels of several mediators of chronic low-grade inflammation (Handschin and Spiegelman 2008), which increase with sedentary habits. This kind of sustained, unresolved, low-grade sterile inflammation has been linked to the etiology of many diseases such as diabetes, cancer, and depression. In this context, the discovery that trained muscle can actively participate in the catabolism of neurotoxic tryptophan metabolites with known deleterious effects on mental health (Agudelo et al. 2014) has added another layer of complexity to the many functions of exercised muscle.

The PGC-1α Family of Transcriptional Coactivators in Skeletal Muscle

Although our understanding of the mechanisms that regulate skeletal muscle adaptation to different exercise challenges remains incomplete, PGC-1α coactivators have been shown to play important roles in this process. These proteins are expressed in energy-demanding tissues such as heart, skeletal muscle, adipose tissue, and brain (Correia et al. 2015). Interestingly, the PGC-1α gene can be transcribed from alternative promoters and its transcripts can be spliced to generate several PGC-1α variants with different biological activities (Martínez-Redondo et al. 2015; Ruas et al. 2012). The expression of PGC-1α1 [the founding member of the family (Puigserver et al. 1998)] is increased by aerobic exercise and regulates genes involved in mitochondrial biogenesis, adaptive thermogenesis, lipid and glucose homeostasis, and fiber-type switching, among others (Correia et al. 2015). For these reasons, reduced PGC-1α1 expression in different tissues has been linked to obesity, diabetes, sarcopenia, and neurodegeneration. Conversely, it has been shown that sustained PGC-1α1 expression in mouse skeletal muscle has several beneficial effects. PGC-1α4 is induced by resistance exercise training and promotes skeletal muscle growth and strength. Importantly, transgenic animals with elevated PGC-1α4 levels in skeletal muscle show increased exercise performance and resistance to atrophy and to cancer-induced cachexia (Ruas et al. 2012). Of the many other PGC-1α isoforms (Martínez-Redondo et al. 2015), PGC-1α2 and α3 have been shown to be involved in alternative splicing of their target genes (Martinez-Redondo et al. 2016), but their main biological roles in skeletal muscle remain unknown.

In addition to helping us understand local adaptations in skeletal muscle, PGC-1α coactivators have been used as tools to investigate the distal actions of exercise-induced myokines. This research has been greatly helped by the use of mouse genetic models with tissue-specific gain or loss of PGC-1α function developed to mimic the physiological and pathophysiological situations associated with altered PGC-1α expression (Rowe and Arany 2014). From these efforts, PGCs have been found to regulate the expression of several myokines involved in inflammation (Handschin and Spiegelman 2008), angiogenesis (VEGF; Arany et al. 2008; Chinsomboon et al. 2009), non-shivering thermogenesis (Fndc5/Irisin, Meteorin-like 1, and β-aminoisobutyric acid; Boström et al. 2012; Rao et al. 2014; Roberts et al. 2014), and muscle mass regulation (Myostatin; Ruas et al. 2012). Similarly, the observation that muscle-specific PGC-1α1 transgenic mice (MKC-PGC-1α; Lin et al. 2002) are resistant to developing depressive-like behaviors when exposed to chronic mild stress resulted in the identification of skeletal muscle as an important site for kynurenine (Kyn) detoxification (Agudelo et al. 2014). Kyn and some of its metabolites are known neurotoxic compounds linked to mental health disorders, such as depression and schizophrenia (Cervenka et al. 2017).

The Kyn Pathway of Tryptophan Degradation

Tryptophan (TRP) is an essential amino acid that cannot be synthesized by the human body and must be acquired from diet. TRP is taken up through the large neutral amino acid transporter (LAT) isoforms 1 to 4, which are also responsible for the uptake of other amino acids such as phenylalanine, tyrosine, and cysteine, and others. However, with the exception of the blood-brain barrier (BBB), LATs have sufficient capacity to avoid significant competition between TRP and other amino acids. A large fraction of plasma TRP circulates bound to albumin and is thus not available for cellular uptake and usage, since only free TRP is taken up by LATs. Under normal circumstances, only about 1% of absorbed TRP is used in protein synthesis, 4–5% is used in the production of the neurotransmitter serotonin and the hormone melatonin, and about 95% is catabolized by the Kyn pathway of TRP degradation (KP). The KP generates NAD^+ as an end-product (mainly in liver and kidney; Houtkooper et al. 2010) and a collection of intermediary metabolites with diverse biological activities (Fig. 1), which have been mainly studied in the context of psychiatric disease.

There are two isozymes that catalyze the first step of TRP degradation: tryptophan 2,3-dioxygenase (TDO) and indoleamine 2,3-dioxygenase (IDO). TDO is specific for TRP and has a more restricted expression pattern (highest in the liver; Yu et al. 2016), whereas IDO is more ubiquitous and metabolizes any compound with

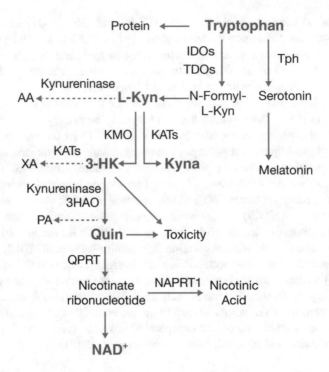

Fig. 1 The kynurenine pathway of tryptophan degradation. *Tph* tryptophan hydroxylase, *IDO* indoleamine 2,3-dioxygenase, *TDO* tryptophan 2,3-dioxygenase, *L-Kyn* L-kynurenine, *AA* Anthranilic acid, *KMO* Kynurenine 3-Monooxygenase, *KATs* Kynurenine amino-transferases, *3HAO* 3-Hydroxyanthranilate 3,4-Dioxygenase, *PA* Picolinic acid, *Quin* Quinolinic acid, *QPRT* Quinolinate phosphoribosyltransferase, *NAD+* Nicotinamide adenine dinucleotide, *NAPRT1* Nicotinate phosphoribosyltransferase

an indol ring structure. The expression and activity of TDO are regulated by cues that include tryptophan, glucocorticoid, and estrogen levels (Yu et al. 2016) and are inhibited under pro-inflammatory conditions. Under those conditions, liver TDO ceases to be the main isozyme responsible for TRP metabolism (normally accounting for 90%), and the extra-hepatic IDO takes on a more prominent role. This shift in TRP metabolism causes an increase of Kyn produced by immune cells that express high levels of IDO in an attempt to control the inflammatory environment. Indeed, as pro-inflammatory cytokines stimulate IDO activity, rising Kyn levels activate the aryl hydrocarbon receptor (AhR) in discrete immune populations and reduce the activity of natural killer cells (NKT), dendritic cells (DC), and T-cells while allowing for Treg proliferation. The net result of this process is an increase in immune tolerance. In line with this, some tumor cells express high IDO/TDO levels as a strategy for escaping the immune system (Platten et al. 2015). Importantly, not all cells possess the complete enzymatic machinery to fully convert TRP to NAD+. In general, the metabolites generated by the KP depend on which enzymes are expressed in each cell type. For example, Kyn aminotransferases (KATs), of which there are four genes in the human genome, are responsible for metabolizing Kyn to kynurenic acid (Kyna) and 3-hydroxykynurenine (3-HK) to xanthurenic acid (XA) (Fig. 1). This is particularly important in the brain, as both Kyna or XA have neuro-protective properties as opposed to several of the downstream metabolites of the KP.

KP Metabolites and Mental Health

The link between the KP and central nervous system (CNS) toxicity has been appreciated for a long time (Lapin 1978). However, it was only in the early 1980s that quinolinic acid (QA) was shown to be a NMDAR agonist (Stone and Perkins 1981), thus providing the first mechanism for KP-induced CNS toxicity. The majority of Kyn reaches the brain from the periphery, as it can easily cross the BBB. However, Kyn can also be produced locally from TRP by astrocytes and microglial cells (Guillemin et al. 2001; Stone and Darlington 2002). Interestingly, although Kyn accumulation in the CNS is consistently associated with neuroinflammation and negative outcomes, its precise mechanism of action remains elusive. In fact, activation of astrocytic AhR (for which Kyn is an agonist) has been shown to be anti-inflammatory in the context of multiple sclerosis (Rothhammer et al. 2016). To date, KP-associated toxicity is mostly understood as the balance between the excitotoxic actions of QA and the neuroprotective effect of Kyna as a NMDAR and α7-nicotinic acetylcholine receptor (α7-nAChR) antagonist. Microglial cells can produce QA whereas astrocytes preferentially generate Kyna (although they can produce QA from extracellular 3-HK, which increases with neuroinflammation). Interestingly, elevated Kyna levels have been found in the cerebrospinal fluid of schizophrenic patients (Linderholm et al. 2012). Conversely, reducing brain Kyna levels in pre-clinical studies (using a KAT2 inhibitor) resulted in improved cognitive function during chemically induced challenges to working and spatial memory tasks (Kozak et al. 2014). In this situation, the pathological consequences of high Kyna concentrations are likely to manifest due to hypoglutamatergic function. 3-HK induces neuronal apoptosis through free-radical generation (Okuda et al. 1998; Polyzos and Ketelhuth 2015). Several metabolites of the pathway have also been linked to neurodegenerative diseases such as Alzheimer's disease, Huntington's disease, Parkinson's disease, among others.

Crosstalk Between Physical Exercise and KP Metabolites

The importance of TRP in exercise has been extensively investigated (Newsholme and Blomstrand 2006), not only due to its critical role in protein synthesis but also in efforts to understand the development of central fatigue and the interplay between diet, exercise, and mood disorders. For example, the increase in circulating free fatty acids that occurs during endurance exercise displaces TRP from albumin and increases free TRP levels, resulting in higher TRP uptake and metabolism in different tissues, with direct impact on the KP. Accordingly, an increase in free TRP plasma levels is followed by an increase in TRP and some of its metabolites in several brain regions associated with the control of mood and fatigue (Blomstrand et al. 1989; Newsholme and Blomstrand 2006).

High TRP uptake during exercise could lead to higher NAD^+ production, which is indeed increased in tissues such as the liver (which is able to fully catabolize TRP). However, the risk of accumulating KP metabolites that can cross the BBB (e.g., Kyn and 3-HK) could have detrimental effects. Recently, it has been shown that exercise increases the expression of KAT enzymes in skeletal muscle (Agudelo et al. 2014; Schlittler et al. 2016), promoting the conversion of Kyn into Kyna, which does not cross the BBB (Agudelo et al. 2014). Peripheral Kyn catabolism prevents its accumulation in the brain and the associated deleterious effects. This is particularly relevant in the context of stress-induced depression, which is characterized by high Kyn levels. This work has provided a mechanism for how physical exercise can improve mental health. Exercise training activates muscle KAT expression and Kyn detoxification by inducing the expression of PGC-1α1 and the PPARα/δ transcription factors, which offers potential therapeutic targets for future antidepressant medications. Interestingly, elevated NAD^+ levels could further promote this mechanism, as NAD+ is a positive regulator of Sirtuin1, which in turn activates PGC-1α1 through lysine deacetylation (Rodgers et al. 2005). Sirtuins have multiple effects on the regulation of cellular energy metabolism, metabolic enzymes and oxidative stress responses in mitochondria (Cantó et al. 2015). Therefore, alterations in the KP may ultimately affect skeletal muscle metabolism and function through multiple concurrent mechanisms.

Future Perspectives and Considerations

TRP is without doubt an important player in many critical functions of a living organism. In addition to being a building block for protein synthesis, TRP plays a role in mental health, energy homeostasis, and immune regulation. It is exciting to see research in these different areas becoming more and more interdisciplinary.

Although we have focused here mainly on post-absorptive TRP metabolism, this amino acid can be sequestered by gut microbiota and converted to tryptamine (Williams et al. 2014) or other indole compounds such as indole-3-propionic acid and indole-3-aldehyde (Rothhammer et al. 2016). Indol compounds serve as important signals between bacteria and between bacteria and their host. Indols are also AhR agonists involved in the local immunomodulation of host tolerance responses and, distally, in the regulation of CNS inflammation (Hubbard et al. 2015). It is therefore critical to consider the effect of the microbiome on TRP metabolism and host physiology. For example, germ-free (GF) mice show reduced anxiety-like behavior, and this phenotype is reversed after colonization. This observation suggests that gut-derived molecules can modulate mood and possibly cognition, and it opens interesting challenges in the discovery of novel pathways of gut-brain communication (Heijtz et al. 2011). Physical exercise also has an impact on gut microbiome composition, but it remains to be explored if this directly impacts on gut TRP metabolism.

The KP is highly conserved evolutionarily, which allows for its study in simpler organisms to dissect its many functions. For example, Kyna has been shown to be involved in *C. elegans* feeding behavior in a NMDAR-dependent mechanism (Lemieux et al. 2015). It will be interesting to continue exploring the role of KP metabolites as possible mediators of inter-organ communication, which could integrate nutrition, metabolism, and immune responses, with all the physiological and pathophysiological implications this could have.

Acknowledgments The authors wish to acknowledge members of the Ruas lab for critical reading of the manuscript and funding from the Swedish Research Council, the Novo Nordisk Foundation (Denmark), Karolinska Institutet, The Lars Hierta Memorial Foundation, The Strategic Research Program (SRP) in Diabetes, and The SRP in Regenerative Medicine at Karolinska Institutet.

References

Agudelo LZ, Femenía T, Orhan F, Porsmyr-Palmertz M, Goiny M, Martinez-Redondo V, Correia JC, Izadi M, Bhat M, Schuppe-Koistinen I, Pettersson AT, Ferreira DM, Krook A, Barres R, Zierath JR, Erhardt S, Lindskog M, Ruas JL (2014) Skeletal muscle PGC-1α1 modulates kynurenine metabolism and mediates resilience to stress-induced depression. Cell 159:33–45

Arany Z, Foo S-Y, Ma Y, Ruas JL, Bommi-Reddy A, Girnun G, Cooper M, Laznik D, Chinsomboon J, Rangwala SM, Baek KH, Rosenzweig A, Spiegelman BM (2008) HIF-independent regulation of VEGF and angiogenesis by the transcriptional coactivator PGC-1a. Nat Lett 451:1008–1013

Blomstrand E, Perrett D, Parry-Billings M, Newsholme E (1989) Effect of sustained exercise on plasma amino acid concentrations and on 5-hydroxytryptamine metabolism in six different brain regions in the rat. Acta Physiol Scand 136:473–481

Boström P, Wu J, Jedrychowski MP, Korde A, Ye L, Lo JC, Rasbach KA, Boström EA, Choi JH, Long JZ, Kajimura S, Zingaretti MC, Vind BF, Tu H, Cinti S, Højlund K, Gygi SP, Spiegelman BM (2012) A PGC1-α-dependent myokine that drives brown-fat-like development of white fat and thermogenesis. Nature 48:463–468

Cantó C, Menzies KJ, Auwerx J (2015) NAD+ metabolism and the control of energy homeostasis: a balancing act between mitochondria and the nucleus. Cell Metab 22:31–53

Cervenka I, Agudelo LZ, Ruas JL (2017) Kynurenines: tryptophan's fantastic metabolites in exercise, inflammation, and mental health. Science (in press)

Chinsomboon J, Ruas J, Gupta RK, Thom R, Shoag J, Rowe GC, Sawada N, Raghuram S, Arany Z (2009) The transcriptional coactivator PGC-1α mediates exercise-induced angiogenesis in skeletal muscle. Proc Natl Acad Sci 106:21401–21406

Cooper C, Moon HY, van Praag H (2017) On the run for hippocampal plasticity. Cold Spring Harb Perspect Med a029736

Correia JC, Ferreira DMS, Ruas JL (2015) Intercellular: local and systemic actions of skeletal muscle PGC-1s. Trends Endocrinol Metab 26:305–314

Giudice J, Taylor JM (2017) Muscle as a paracrine and endocrine organ. Curr Opin Pharmacol 34:49–55

Guillemin GJ, Kerr SJ, Smythe GA, Smith DGN, Kapoor V, Armati PJ, Croitoru J, Brew BJ (2001) Kynurenine pathway metabolism in human astrocytes: a paradox for neuronal protection. J Neurochem 78:842–853

Handschin C, Spiegelman BM (2008) The role of exercise and PGC1α in inflammation and chronic disease. Nature 454:463–469

Hawley JA (2004) Exercise as a therapeutic intervention for the prevention and treatment of insulin resistance. Diabetes Metab Res Rev 20:383–393

Hawley JA, Hargreaves M, Joyner MJ, Zierath JR (2014) Integrative biology of exercise. Cell 159:738–749

Heijtz RD, Wang S, Anuar F, Qian Y, Bjorkholm B, Samuelsson A, Hibberd ML, Forssberg H, Pettersson S (2011) Normal gut microbiota modulates brain development and behavior. Proc Natl Acad Sci 108:3047–3052

Houtkooper RH, Canto C, Wanders RJ, Auwerx J (2010) The secret life of NAD+: an old metabolite controlling new metabolic signaling pathways. Endocr Rev 31:194–223

Hubbard TD, Murray IA, Perdew GH (2015) Indole and tryptophan metabolism: endogenous and dietary routes to Ah receptor activation. Drug Metab Dispos 43:1522–1535

Kozak R, Campbell BM, Strick CA, Horner W, Hoffmann WE, Kiss T, Chapin DS, McGinnis D, Abbott AL, Roberts BM, Fonseca K, Guanowsky V, Young DA, Seymour PA, Dounay A, Hajos M, Williams GV, Castner SA (2014) Reduction of brain kynurenic acid improves cognitive function. J Neurosci 34:10592–10602

Lapin IP (1978) Stimulant and convulsive effects of kynurenines injected into brain ventricles in mice. J Neural Transm 42:37–43

Lemieux GA, Cunningham KA, Lin L, Mayer F, Werb Z, Ashrafi K (2015) Kynurenic acid is a nutritional cue that enables behavioral plasticity. Cell 160:119–131

Lin J, Wu H, Tarr PT, Zhang C-Y, Wu Z, Boss O, Michael LF, Puigserver P, Isotani E, Olson EN, Lowell BB, Bassel-Duby R, Spiegelman BM (2002) Transcriptional co-activator PGC-1 a drives the formation of slow-twitch muscle fibre. Nature 418:797–801

Linderholm KR, Skogh E, Olsson SK, Dahl ML, Holtze M, Engberg G, Samuelsson M, Erhardt S (2012) Increased levels of kynurenine and kynurenic acid in the CSF of patients with schizophrenia. Schizophr Bull 38:426–432

Martínez-Redondo V, Pettersson AT, Ruas JL (2015) The hitchhiker's guide to PGC-1a isoform structure and biological functions. Diabetologia 58:1969–1977

Martinez-Redondo V, Jannig PR, Correia JC, Ferreira DMS, Cervenka I, Lindvall JM, Sinha I, Izadi M, Pettersson-Klein AT, Agudelo LZ, Gimenez-Cassina A, Brum PC, Dahlman-Wright K, Ruas J (2016) Peroxisome proliferator-activated receptor gamma coactivator-1a isoforms selectively regulate multiple splicing events on target genes. J Biol Chem 291:15169–15184

Newsholme EA, Blomstrand E (2006) Branched-chain amino acids and central fatigue. J Nutr 136:274–276

Okuda S, Nishiyama N, Saito H, Katsuki H (1998) 3-Hydroxykynurenine, an endogenous oxidative stress generator, causes neuronal cell death with apoptotic features and region selectivity. J Neurochem 70:299–307

Platten M, von Knebel Doeberitz N, Oezen I, Wick W, Ochs K (2015) Cancer immunotherapy by targeting IDO1/TDO and their downstream effectors. Front Immunol 6:1–7

Polyzos KA, Ketelhuth DFJ (2015) The role of the kynurenine pathway of tryptophan metabolism in cardiovascular disease. Hamostaseologie 35:128–136

Puigserver P, Wu Z, Park CW, Graves R, Wright M, Spiegelman BM (1998) A cold-inducible coactivator of nuclear receptors linked to adaptive thermogenesis. Cell 92:829–839

Rao RR, Long JZ, White JP, Svensson KJ, Lou J, Lokurkar I, Jedrychowski MP, Ruas JL, Wrann CD, Lo JC, Camera DM, Lachey J, Gygi S, Seehra J, Hawley JA, Spiegelman BM (2014) Meteorin-like is a hormone that regulates immune-adipose Iinteractions to increase beige fat thermogenesis. Cell 157:1279–1291

Roberts LD, Bostrom P, O'Sullivan JF, Schinzel RT, Lewis GD, Dejam A, Lee Y-K, Palma MJ, Calhoun S, Georgiadi A, Chen MH, Ramachandran VS, Larson MG, Bouchard C, Rankinen T,

Souza AL, Clish CB, Wang TJ, Estall JL, Soukas AA, Cowan CA, Spiegelman BM, Gerszten RE (2014) Beta-aminoisobutyric acid induces browning of white fat and hepatic beta-oxidation and is inversely correlated with cardiometabolic risk factors. Cell Metab 19:96–108

Rodgers JT, Lerin C, Haas W, Gygi SP, Spiegelman BM, Puigserver P (2005) Nutrient control of glucose homeostasis through a complex of PGC-1a and SIRT1. Nature 434:113–118

Rothhammer V, Mascanfroni ID, Bunse L, Takenaka MC, Kenison JE, Mayo L, Chao C-C, Patel B, Yan R, Blain M, Alvarez JI, Kébir H, Anandasabapathy N, Izquierdo G, Jung S, Obholzer N, Pochet N, Clish CB, Prinz M, Prat A, Antel J, Quintana FJ (2016) Type I interferons and microbial metabolites of tryptophan modulate astrocyte activity and central nervous system inflammation via the aryl hydrocarbon receptor. Nat Med 22:586–597

Rowe GC, Arany Z (2014) Genetic models of PGC-1 and glucose metabolism and homeostasis. Rev Endocr Metab Disord 15:21–29

Ruas JL, White JP, Rao RR, Kleiner S, Brannan KT, Harrison BC, Greene NP, Wu J, Estall JL, Irving BA, Lanza IR, Rasbach KA, Okutsu M, Nair KS, Yan Z, Leinwand LA, Spiegelman BM (2012) A PGC-1α isoform induced by resistance training regulates skeletal muscle hypertrophy. Cell 151:1319–1331

Schlittler M, Goiny M, Agudelo LZ, Venckunas T, Brazaitis M, Skurvydas A, Kamandulis S, Ruas JL, Erhardt S, Westerblad H, Andersson DC (2016) Endurance exercise increases skeletal muscle kynurenine aminotransferases and plasma kynurenic acid in humans. Am J Physiol Cell Physiol 310:C836–C840

Stone TW, Darlington LG (2002) Endogenous kynurenines as targets for drug discovery and development. Nat Rev Drug Discov 1:609–620

Stone TW, Perkins MN (1981) Quinolinic acid: a potent endogenous excitant at amino acid receptors in CNS. Eur J Pharmacol 72:411–412

Williams BB, Van Benschoten AH, Cimermancic P, Donia MS, Zimmermann M, Taketani M, Ishihara A, Kashyap PC, Fraser JS, Fischbach MA (2014) Discovery and characterization of gut microbiota decarboxylases that can produce the neurotransmitter tryptamine. Cell Host Microbe 16:495–503

Yu CP, Pan ZZ, Luo DY (2016) TDO as a therapeutic target in brain diseases. Metab Brain Dis 31:737–747

The Role of FNDC5/Irisin in the Nervous System and as a Mediator for Beneficial Effects of Exercise on the Brain

Mohammad Rashedul Islam, Michael F. Young, and Christiane D. Wrann

Abstract Exercise can improve cognitive function and the outcome of neurode-generative diseases like Alzheimer's disease. This effect has been linked to the increased expression of brain-derived neurotrophic factor (BDNF). However, the underlying molecular mechanisms driving the elevation of this neurotrophin remain unknown. Recently, we have reported a PGC-1α-FNDC5/irisin pathway that is activated by exercise in the hippocampus in mice and induces a neuroprotective gene program, including *Bdnf*. This review will focus on FNDC5 and its secreted form "irisin," a newly discovered myokine, its role in the nervous system and its therapeutic potential. In addition, we will briefly discuss the role of other exercise-induced myokines in positive brain effects.

Introduction

Exercise, especially endurance exercise, is known to have beneficial effects on brain health and cognitive function (Cotman et al. 2007; Mattson 2012; Voss et al. 2013). This improvement in cognitive function with exercise has been most prominently observed in the aging population (Colcombe and Kramer 2003). Exercise has also been reported to ameliorate outcomes in neurological diseases such as depression, epilepsy, stroke, and Alzheimer's and Parkinson's disease (Ahlskog 2011; Arida et al. 2008; Buchman et al. 2012; Russo-Neustadt et al. 1999; Zhang et al. 2012). The effects of exercise on the brain are most apparent in the hippocampus and the dentate gyrus, a part of the brain involved in learning and memory. Specific beneficial effects of exercise in the brain have been reported to include increases in the size of, and blood flow to, the hippocampus in humans and morphological changes in dendrites and dendritic spines, increased synapse plasticity and, importantly, de novo neurogenesis in the dentate gyrus in various mouse models of exercise (Cotman

M. R. Islam • M. F. Young • C. D. Wrann (✉)
Massachussetts General Hospital and Harvard Medical School, Charlestown, MA, USA
e-mail: cwrann@mgh.harvard.edu

© The Author(s) 2017
B. Spiegelman (ed.), *Hormones, Metabolism and the Benefits of Exercise*,
Research and Perspectives in Endocrine Interactions,
https://doi.org/10.1007/978-3-319-72790-5_8

et al. 2007; Mattson 2012). De novo neurogenesis in the adult brain is observed in only two areas; the dentate gyrus of the hippocampus is one of them. Exercise is one of the few known stimuli of this de novo neurogenesis (Kobilo et al. 2011).

One important molecular mediator of these beneficial responses in the brain to exercise is the induction of neurotrophins/growth factors, most notably brain-derived neurotrophic factor (BDNF). In animal models, BDNF is induced in various regions of the brain with exercise, most robustly in the hippocampus (Cotman et al. 2007). BDNF promotes many aspects of brain development, including neuronal cell survival, differentiation, migration, dendritic arborization, synaptogenesis and plasticity (Greenberg et al. 2009; Park and Poo 2013). In addition, BDNF is essential for synaptic plasticity, hippocampal function, and learning (Kuipers and Bramham 2006). Highlighting the relevance of BDNF in humans, individuals carrying the Val66Met mutation in the *Bdnf* gene exhibit decreased secretion of BDNF, decreased volume of specific brain regions, deficits in episodic memory function and increased anxiety and depression (Egan et al. 2003; Hariri et al. 2003). Blocking BDNF signaling with anti-TrkB antibodies attenuates the exercise-induced improvement of acquisition and retention of a spatial learning task, as well as the exercise-induced expression of synaptic proteins (Vaynman et al. 2004, 2006). However, the underlying mechanism that induces BDNF in exercise remains incompletely understood.

We recently described a role for the newly discovered "exercise-hormone," FNDC5 (Bostrom et al. 2012), and its secreted form, "irisin," in the protective effects of exercise on the brain. *Fndc5* expression is induced by exercise in the hippocampus in mice; it can, in turn, activate BDNF and other neuroprotective genes (Wrann et al. 2013). Importantly, peripheral delivery of FNDC5 to the liver via adenoviral vectors, resulting in elevated blood irisin, induces expression of *Bdnf* and other neuroprotective genes in the hippocampus. These data indicate that either irisin itself can cross the blood-brain-barrier to induce gene expression changes or irisin induces a "factor x" that can, which has significant implications for irisin as a novel therapeutic target. This review will examine previous literature about FNDC5/irisin as well as its therapeutic potential for treating neurodegenerative disease.

Discovery of FNDC5/Irisin

In 2002, two groups independently cloned a novel gene termed either PeP or, alternatively, Frcp2, that contained a fibronectin type III (FNIII) domain; it is now named FNDC5 (Ferrer-Martinez et al. 2002; Teufel et al. 2002). Recently, our group identified FNDC5 as a PGC-1α-dependent myokine that is secreted from muscle during exercise and induces some major metabolic benefits of exercise (Bostrom et al. 2012).

FNDC5 is a glycosylated type I membrane protein. It contains a N-terminal signal peptide [amino acid (aa) 1-28], a FNIII domain (aa 33–124), a transmembrane domain (aa 150–170), and a cytoplasmic tail (aa 171–209) (www.uniporot.org) (Fig. 1). The secreted form of FNDC5 contains 112 amino acids (aa 29-140), named irisin, and is generated by proteolytic cleavage and is released into the circulation.

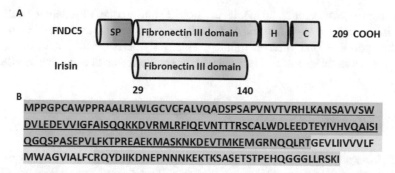

Fig. 1 Analysis of Irisin Peptides by Mass Spectrometry. (**a**) Scheme of the murine FNDC5 protein structure (top) and murine irisin protein structure (bottom). *SP* signal peptide, *H* hydrophobic domain, *C* cytoplasmic domain. (**b**) Murine FNDC5 amino acid sequence with corresponding domains colored. The irisin sequence is underlined

The protease/sheddase responsible for that cleavage has not yet been identified. Irisin has been crystallized and its structure has been solved (Schumacher et al. 2013). Interestingly, the FNIII-like domain shows an unusual confirmation, with a continuous intersubunit beta-sheet dimer, that has not been previously described for any other FNIII protein. Subsequent biochemical experiments confirmed the existence of irisin (bacterial recombinant) as a homodimer.

Irisin in Humans

Irisin is a highly conserved polypeptide across mammals and is, in fact, 100% identical in mice and humans (Bostrom et al. 2012). Such a high degree of conservation is often the result of evolutionary pressure to conserve function. Interestingly, the human FNDC5 has an atypical start of translation, ATA in place of ATG, as compared to mouse Fndc5. While it is now known that a few percent of eukaryotic mRNAs begin translation with non-ATG start codons (Ingolia et al. 2011; Ivanov et al. 2011; Peabody 1989) and are often associated with regulation on the translational level (Chang and Wang 2004; Starck et al. 2012), recent reports (Albrecht et al. 2015, Raschke et al. 2013) have argued that this ATA codon in human FNDC5 was a "null mutation" or a "myth" and, as a result, human irisin would not be produced. Furthermore, many reports from other groups measuring irisin in humans by Western blot or ELISA have suggested results to be artefacts of poor antibody specificity (Albrecht et al. 2015; Erickson 2013; Raschke et al. 2013), even though an earlier study had detected irisin circulating in human plasma using mass spectrometry, an unbiased method independent of the quality of existing antibodies (Jedrychowski et al. 2015; Lee et al. 2014). To identify and quantify irisin in human plasma, we used targeted mass spectrometry with control peptides enriched with stable isotopes as internal standards. This precise, state-of-the-art method demonstrated that human irisin was mainly translated from its non-canonical ATA start codon (Jedrychowski et al. 2015). In addition, it showed that, in sedentary individuals, irisin circulated at ~3.6 ng/ml and that it was significantly increased in individuals undergoing aerobic interval training. This study determined that, at the atomic level, human irisin exists, and is regulated by certain forms of aerobic exercise.

FNDC5/Irisin in Exercise

FNDC5/irisin was first described as an exercise-induced myokine by Bostrom et al. in 2012, where they observed upregulation of *Fndc5* gene expression in skeletal muscle and increased serum irisin levels after prolonged endurance exercise in both mice and humans. Increasing the circulating levels of irisin by overexpression of FNDC5 from adenoviral vectors in the liver led to an increase in "browning" of the white inguinal adipose tissue, i.e., the upregulation of mitochondrial gene expression, especially of *Ucp1*, and an increased glucose tolerance in mice. Both are among the major metabolic benefits of endurance exercise. By now, there are around 50 published papers that investigate the role of FNDC5 and/or irisin in exercise, including both rodent studies and clinical trials in humans. Induction of *Fndc5* mRNA in skeletal muscle by endurance exercise has been confirmed in several studies in both mice (Quinn et al. 2015; Tiano et al. 2015; Wrann et al. 2013) and humans (Albrecht et al. 2015; Lecker et al. 2012; Norheim et al. 2014) using qPCR or RNA sequencing. As with all clinical studies, there are a lot of variables to consider, such as retrospective studies vs. interventional trials, age and fitness level of the subjects and, most importantly, the type of exercise protocol used and time point of sampling. However, a consensus is building, supported by studies that reported positive associations between irisin plasma level and exercise, performed early sampling and high intensity training protocols levels (Daskalopoulou et al. 2014; Huh et al. 2014; Kraemer et al. 2014; Malcolm Eaton et al. 2017; Norheim et al. 2014). Plasma levels of irisin and BDNF have been shown to be positively correlated with cognitive function in endurance athletes (Belviranli et al. 2016).

The brief rise in circulating irisin levels after exercise is suggestive of an acute shedding event of irisin during exercise. There is little to no evidence thus far that FNDC5 or irisin is upregulated by resistance exercise in mouse or human This is not unexpected, since endurance exercise activates PGC-1α1, which has been shown to be the upstream regulator of Fndc5 gene expression, whereas resistance exercise activates a different isoform of PGC-1α1, PGC-1α4 (Ruas et al. 2012).

FNDC5/Irisin in Neuronal Development

Fndc5 is highly expressed in the brain, including the Purkinje cells of the cerebellum (Dun et al. 2013; Ferrer-Martinez et al. 2002; Teufel et al. 2002). Irisin, the shed form of FNDC5, was identified in human cerebrospinal fluid by Western blot (Piya et al. 2014). In addition, immunoreactivity against the extracellular domain of FNDC5/irisin was detected in human hypothalamic sections, especially paraventricular neurons (Piya et al. 2014). Other tissues with high FNDC5 levels include skeletal muscle and the heart. *Fndc5* gene expression increases during differentiation of rat pheochromocytoma-derived PC12 cells into neuron-like cells (Ostadsharif et al. 2011). FNDC5 levels are enhanced after the differentiation of human embryonic stem cell-derived neural cells into neurons (Ghahrizjani et al. 2015) as well as during the maturation of primary cortical neurons in culture and during brain development in vivo (Wrann et al. 2013).

Knockdown of FNDC5 in neuronal precursors impaired their development into mature neurons (and astrocytes), suggesting a developmental role for FNDC5 in neurons (Hashemi et al. 2013). Despite this finding, forced expression of FNDC5 during neuronal precursor formation from mouse embryonic stem cells increased mature neuronal markers (Map2, b-tubulinIII and Neurocan) and an astrocyte marker (GFAP) and BDNF. However, overexpression of FNDC5 in undifferentiated mouse embryonic stem cells did not have these effects, indicating that FNDC5 supports neural differentiation rather than lineage commitment (Forouzanfar et al. 2015). Pharmacological doses of recombinant irisin increased cell proliferation in the mouse H19-7 hippocampal cell line (Moon et al. 2013). Furthermore, forced expression of FNDC5 in primary cortical neurons increased cell survival in culture, whereas knockdown of FNDC5 had the opposite effect (Wrann et al. 2013).

FNDC5/Irisin: Other Effects in the CNS

The group of Dr. Mulholland (University of Michigan) had taken in interest in the central nervous effects of irisin. In a first study, they injected irisin either into third ventricle of rats or intravenously measured the effects on blood pressure and cardiac contractibility (Zhang et al. 2015a). Central administration of irisin activated neurons in the paraventricular nuclei of the hypothalamus, as indicated by increased c-fos immunoreactivity. Central irisin administration also increased both blood pressure and cardiac contractibility. In contrast, i.v. injection of irisin reduced blood pressure in both control and spontaneously hypertensive rats. In a second study, Zhang et al. showed that central treatment of rats with irisin-Fc led to an increase in physical activity as measured as total travel distance, ambulatory counts and time, and vertical counts and time compared to control animals receiving IgG Fc peptide (Zhang et al. 2015b). In addition, the centrally applied irisin also induced significant increases in oxygen consumption, carbon dioxide production and heat production, indicating an increase in metabolic activity- possibly through SNS activation. Similarly, intra-hypothalamic injection of irisin decreased food intake in rats possibly by stimulating anorexigenic peptides and inhibiting dopamine, norepinephrine and orexin-A (Ferrante et al. 2016).

A recent study investigated the neuroprotective potential of irisin treatments in cerebral ischemia. Irisin improved survival of cultured PC12 neuronal cells in oxygen glucose deprivation. I.v. injection of recombinant irisin reduced brain infarct and edema volume and improved the neurological score in MCAO stroke model (Li et al. 2017). Systemic irisin administration has also been shown to ameliorate depressive-like behavior in a chronic unpredictable stress model in rats (Wang and Pan 2016).

Exercise Induces Hippocampal BDNF Through a PGC-1α/FNDC5 Pathway

In a recent study, we have shown that FNDC5 is also elevated in the hippocampus of mice undergoing endurance exercise regimen of 30-days free-wheel running. Neuronal *Fndc5* gene expression is regulated by PGC-1α and Pgc1a$^{-/-}$ mice show reduced *Fndc5* expression in the brain. Forced expression of FNDC5 in primary cortical neurons increases *Bdnf* expression, whereas RNAi-mediated knockdown of FNDC5 reduces *Bdnf*. Importantly, peripheral delivery of FNDC5 to the liver via adenoviral vectors, resulting in elevated blood irisin, induces expression of *Bdnf* and other neuroprotective genes in the hippocampus. Taken together, our findings link endurance exercise and the important metabolic mediators, PGC-1α and FNDC5, with BDNF expression in the brain. Interestingly, a recent study investigating the effects of the flavonoid quercetin hypobaric hypoxia, reported that quercetin administration to hyperbaric hypoxic rats increased expression of PGC-1α, FNDC5, and BDNF in the hippocampus (Liu et al. 2015). While more research will be required to determine whether the FNDC5/irisin protein can improve cognitive function in animals, this study suggests that a hormone administered peripherally could induce some of the effects of endurance exercise on the brain (Fig. 2).

Other Circulating Factors from the Muscle

While FNDC5/irisin is a very interesting molecule that holds therapeutic promise, this is not to say that we think that FNDC5/irisin captures all the benefits of exercise on the brain or that is the only important secreted molecule from muscle in exercise. In fact, other such molecules have been described, including BDNF, IGF-1, and VEGF, kynurenic acid, cathepsin B, as well as a variety of cytokines and chemokines, to name a few (Agudelo et al. 2014; Moon et al. 2016; Phillips et al. 2014; Voss et al. 2013). We expect that in the future, additional molecules will be discovered and some may reach their full therapeutic potential.

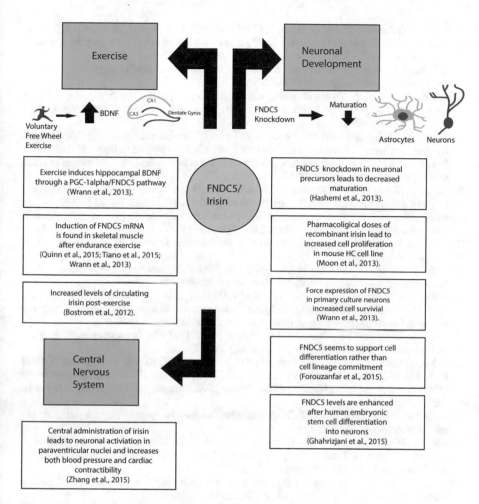

Fig. 2 Summary of FNDC5/irisin effects on the brain

Acknowledgements This work was supported by the NIH (NS087096). I also thank Dr. Mark Jedrychowski for support with the art work.

References

Agudelo LZ, Femenia T, Orhan F, Porsmyr-Palmertz M, Goiny M, Martinez-Redondo V, Correia JC, Izadi M, Bhat M, Schuppe-Koistinen I, Pettersson AT, Ferreira DM, Krook A, Barres R, Zierath JR, Erhardt S, Lindskog M, Ruas JL (2014) Skeletal muscle PGC-1alpha1 modulates kynurenine metabolism and mediates resilience to stress-induced depression. Cell 159:33–45

Ahlskog JE (2011) Does vigorous exercise have a neuroprotective effect in Parkinson disease? Neurology 77:288–294

Albrecht E, Norheim F, Thiede B, Holen T, Ohashi T, Schering L, Lee S, Brenmoehl J, Thomas S, Drevon CA, Erickson HP, Maak S (2015) Irisin – a myth rather than an exercise-inducible myokine. Sci Rep 5:8889

Arida RM, Cavalheiro EA, da Silva AC, Scorza FA (2008) Physical activity and epilepsy: proven and predicted benefits. Sports Med 38:607–615

Belviranli M, Okudan N, Kabak B, Erdogan M, Karanfilci M (2016) The relationship between brain-derived neurotrophic factor, irisin and cognitive skills of endurance athletes. Phys Sportsmed 44:290–296

Bostrom P, Wu J, Jedrychowski MP, Korde A, Ye L, Lo JC, Rasbach KA, Bostrom EA, Choi JH, Long JZ, Kajimura S, Zingaretti MC, Vind BF, Tu H, Cinti S, Højlund K, Gygi SP, Spiegelman BM (2012) A PGC1-alpha-dependent myokine that drives brown-fat-like development of white fat and thermogenesis. Nature 481:463–468

Buchman AS, Boyle PA, Yu L, Shah RC, Wilson RS, Bennett DA (2012) Total daily physical activity and the risk of AD and cognitive decline in older adults. Neurology 78:1323–1329

Chang KJ, Wang CC (2004) Translation initiation from a naturally occurring non-AUG codon in Saccharomyces cerevisiae. J Biol Chem 279:13778–13785

Colcombe S, Kramer AF (2003) Fitness effects on the cognitive function of older adults: a meta-analytic study. Psychol Sci 14:125–130

Cotman CW, Berchtold NC, Christie LA (2007) Exercise builds brain health: key roles of growth factor cascades and inflammation. Trends Neurosci 30:464–472

Daskalopoulou SS, Cooke AB, Gomez YH, Mutter AF, Filippaios A, Mesfum ET, Mantzoros CS (2014) Plasma irisin levels progressively increase in response to increasing exercise workloads in young, healthy, active subjects. Eur J Endocrinol 171:343–352

Dun SL, Lyu RM, Chen YH, Chang JK, Luo JJ, Dun NJ (2013) Irisin-immunoreactivity in neural and non-neural cells of the rodent. Neuroscience 240:155–162

Egan MF, Kojima M, Callicott JH, Goldberg TE, Kolachana BS, Bertolino A, Zaitsev E, Gold B, Goldman D, Dean M, Lu B, Weinberger DR (2003) The BDNF val66met polymorphism affects activity-dependent secretion of BDNF and human memory and hippocampal function. Cell 112:257–269

Erickson HP (2013) Irisin and FNDC5 in retrospect: an exercise hormone or a transmembrane receptor? Adipocyte 2:289–293

Ferrante C, Orlando G, Recinella L, Leone S, Chiavaroli A, Di Nisio C, Shohreh R, Manippa F, Ricciuti A, Vacca M, Brunetti L (2016) Central inhibitory effects on feeding induced by the adipo-myokine irisin. Eur J Pharmacol 791:389–394

Ferrer-Martinez A, Ruiz-Lozano P, Chien KR (2002) Mouse PeP: a novel peroxisomal protein linked to myoblast differentiation and development. Dev Dyn 224:154–167

Forouzanfar M, Rabiee F, Ghaedi K, Beheshti S, Tanhaei S, Shoaraye Nejati A, Jodeiri Farshbaf M, Baharvand H, Nasr-Esfahani MH (2015) Fndc5 overexpression facilitated neural differentiation of mouse embryonic stem cells. Cell Biol Int 39:629–637

Ghahrizjani FA, Ghaedi K, Salamian A, Tanhaei S, Nejati AS, Salehi H, Nabiuni M, Baharvand H, Nasr-Esfahani MH (2015) Enhanced expression of FNDC5 in human embryonic stem cell-derived neural cells along with relevant embryonic neural tissues. Gene 557:123–129

Greenberg ME, Xu B, Lu B, Hempstead BL (2009) New insights in the biology of BDNF synthesis and release: implications in CNS function. J Neurosci 29:12764–12767

Hariri AR, Goldberg TE, Mattay VS, Kolachana BS, Callicott JH, Egan MF, Weinberger DR (2003) Brain-derived neurotrophic factor val66met polymorphism affects human memory-related hippocampal activity and predicts memory performance. J Neurosci 23:6690–6694

Hashemi MS, Ghaedi K, Salamian A, Karbalaie K, Emadi-Baygi M, Tanhaei S, Nasr-Esfahani MH, Baharvand H (2013) Fndc5 knockdown significantly decreased neural differentiation rate of mouse embryonic stem cells. Neuroscience 231:296–304

Huh JY, Mougios V, Kabasakalis A, Fatouros I, Siopi A, Douroudos II, Filippaios A, Panagiotou G, Park KH, Mantzoros CS (2014) Exercise-induced irisin secretion is independent of age or fitness level and increased irisin may directly modulate muscle metabolism through AMPK activation. J Clin Endocrinol Metab 99:E2154–E2161

Ingolia NT, Lareau LF, Weissman JS (2011) Ribosome profiling of mouse embryonic stem cells reveals the complexity and dynamics of mammalian proteomes. Cell 147:789–802

Ivanov IP, Firth AE, Michel AM, Atkins JF, Baranov PV (2011) Identification of evolutionarily conserved non-AUG-initiated N-terminal extensions in human coding sequences. Nucleic Acids Res 39:4220–4234

Jedrychowski MP, Wrann CD, Paulo JA, Gerber KK, Szpyt J, Robinson MM, Nair KS, Gygi SP, Spiegelman BM (2015) Detection and quantitation of circulating human irisin by tandem mass spectrometry. Cell Metab 22:734–740

Kobilo T, Liu QR, Gandhi K, Mughal M, Shaham Y, van Praag H (2011) Running is the neurogenic and neurotrophic stimulus in environmental enrichment. Learn Mem 18:605–609

Kraemer RR, Shockett P, Webb ND, Shah U, Castracane VD (2014) A transient elevated irisin blood concentration in response to prolonged, moderate aerobic exercise in young men and women. Horm Metab Res 46:150–154

Kuipers SD, Bramham CR (2006) Brain-derived neurotrophic factor mechanisms and function in adult synaptic plasticity: new insights and implications for therapy. Curr Opin Drug Discov Dev 9:580–586

Lecker SH, Zavin A, Cao P, Arena R, Allsup K, Daniels KM, Joseph J, Schulze PC, Forman DE (2012) Expression of the irisin precursor FNDC5 in skeletal muscle correlates with aerobic exercise performance in patients with heart failure. Circ Heart Fail 5:812–818

Lee P, Linderman JD, Smith S, Brychta RJ, Wang J, Idelson C, Perron RM, Werner CD, Phan GQ, Kammula US et al (2014) Irisin and FGF21 are cold-induced endocrine activators of brown fat function in humans. Cell Metab 19:302–309

Li DJ, Li YH, Yuan HB, Qu LF, Wang P (2017) The novel exercise-induced hormone irisin protects against neuronal injury via activation of the Akt and ERK1/2 signaling pathways and contributes to the neuroprotection of physical exercise in cerebral ischemia. Metabolism 68:31–42

Liu P, Zou D, Yi L, Chen M, Gao Y, Zhou R, Zhang Q, Zhou Y, Zhu J, Chen K et al (2015) Quercetin ameliorates hypobaric hypoxia-induced memory impairment through mitochondrial and neuron function adaptation via the PGC-1alpha pathway. Restor Neurol Neurosci 33:143–157

Malcolm Eaton CG, Barry J, Safdar A, Bishop D, Jonathan P (2017) Little impact of a single bout of high-intensity interval exercise and short-term interval training on interleukin-6, FNDC5, and METRNL mRNA expression in human skeletal muscle. J Sport Health Sci 4–0

Mattson MP (2012) Energy intake and exercise as determinants of brain health and vulnerability to injury and disease. Cell Metab 16:706–722

Moon HS, Dincer F, Mantzoros CS (2013) Pharmacological concentrations of irisin increase cell proliferation without influencing markers of neurite outgrowth and synaptogenesis in mouse H19-7 hippocampal cell lines. Metabolism 62:1131–1136

Moon HY, Becke A, Berron D, Becker B, Sah N, Benoni G, Janke E, Lubejko ST, Greig NH, Mattison JA, Duzel E, van Praag H (2016) Running-induced systemic cathepsin B secretion is associated with memory function. Cell Metab 24:332–340

Norheim F, Langleite TM, Hjorth M, Holen T, Kielland A, Stadheim HK, Gulseth HL, Birkeland KI, Jensen J, Drevon CA (2014) The effects of acute and chronic exercise on PGC-1alpha, irisin and browning of subcutaneous adipose tissue in humans. FEBS J 281:739–749

Ostadsharif M, Ghaedi K, Hossein Nasr-Esfahani M, Mojbafan M, Tanhaie S, Karbalaie K, Baharvand H (2011) The expression of peroxisomal protein transcripts increased by retinoic acid during neural differentiation. Differentiation 81:127–132

Park H, Poo MM (2013) Neurotrophin regulation of neural circuit development and function. Nat Rev Neurosci 14:7–23

Peabody DS (1989) Translation initiation at non-AUG triplets in mammalian cells. J Biol Chem 264:5031–5035

Phillips C, Baktir MA, Srivatsan M, Salehi A (2014) Neuroprotective effects of physical activity on the brain: a closer look at trophic factor signaling. Front Cell Neurosci 8:170

Piya MK, Harte AL, Sivakumar K, Tripathi G, Voyias PD, James S, Sabico S, Al-Daghri NM, Saravanan P, Barber TM, Kumar S, Vatish M, McTernan PG (2014) The identification of irisin in human cerebrospinal fluid: influence of adiposity, metabolic markers, and gestational diabetes. Am J Physiol Endocrinol Metab 306:E512–E518

Quinn LS, Anderson BG, Conner JD, Wolden-Hanson T (2015) Circulating irisin levels and muscle FNDC5 mRNA expression are independent of IL-15 levels in mice. Endocrine 50:368–377

Raschke S, Elsen M, Gassenhuber H, Sommerfeld M, Schwahn U, Brockmann B, Jung R, Wisloff U, Tjonna AE, Raastad T, Hallén J, Norheim F, Drevon CA, Romacho T, Eckardt K, Eckel J (2013) Evidence against a beneficial effect of irisin in humans. PLoS One 8:e73680

Ruas JL, White JP, Rao RR, Kleiner S, Brannan KT, Harrison BC, Greene NP, Wu J, Estall JL, Irving BA, Lanza IR, Rasbach KA, Okutsu M, Nair KS, Yan Z, Leinwand LA, Spiegelman BM (2012) A PGC-1alpha isoform induced by resistance training regulates skeletal muscle hypertrophy. Cell 151:1319–1331

Russo-Neustadt A, Beard RC, Cotman CW (1999) Exercise, antidepressant medications, and enhanced brain derived neurotrophic factor expression. Neuropsychopharmacology 21:679–682

Schumacher MA, Chinnam N, Ohashi T, Shah RS, Erickson HP (2013) The structure of irisin reveals a novel intersubunit beta-sheet fibronectin type III (FNIII) dimer: implications for receptor activation. J Biol Chem 288:33738–33744

Starck SR, Jiang V, Pavon-Eternod M, Prasad S, McCarthy B, Pan T, Shastri N (2012) Leucine-tRNA initiates at CUG start codons for protein synthesis and presentation by MHC class I. Science 336:1719–1723

Teufel A, Malik N, Mukhopadhyay M, Westphal H (2002) Frcp1 and Frcp2, two novel fibronectin type III repeat containing genes. Gene 297:79–83

Tiano JP, Springer DA, Rane SG (2015) SMAD3 negatively regulates serum irisin and skeletal muscle FNDC5 and peroxisome proliferator-activated receptor gamma coactivator 1-alpha (PGC-1alpha) during exercise. J Biol Chem 290:7671–7684

Vaynman S, Ying Z, Gomez-Pinilla F (2004) Hippocampal BDNF mediates the efficacy of exercise on synaptic plasticity and cognition. Eur J Neurosci 20:2580–2590

Vaynman SS, Ying Z, Yin D, Gomez-Pinilla F (2006) Exercise differentially regulates synaptic proteins associated to the function of BDNF. Brain Res 1070:124–130

Voss MW, Vivar C, Kramer AF, van Praag H (2013) Bridging animal and human models of exercise-induced brain plasticity. Trends Cogn Sci 17:525–544

Wang S, Pan J (2016) Irisin ameliorates depressive-like behaviors in rats by regulating energy metabolism. Biochem Biophys Res Commun 474:22–28

Wrann CD, White JP, Salogiannnis J, Laznik-Bogoslavski D, Wu J, Ma D, Lin JD, Greenberg ME, Spiegelman BM (2013) Exercise induces hippocampal BDNF through a PGC-1alpha/FNDC5 pathway. Cell Metab 18:649–659

Zhang Q, Wu Y, Zhang P, Sha H, Jia J, Hu Y, Zhu J (2012) Exercise induces mitochondrial biogenesis after brain ischemia in rats. Neuroscience 205:10–17

Zhang W, Chang L, Zhang C, Zhang R, Li Z, Chai B, Li J, Chen E, Mulholland M (2015a) Central and peripheral irisin differentially regulate blood pressure. Cardiovasc Drugs Ther 29:121–127

Zhang W, Chang L, Zhang C, Zhang R, Li Z, Chai B, Li J, Chen E, Mulholland M (2015b) Irisin: a myokine with locomotor activity. Neurosci Lett 595:7–11

Printed in the United States
By Bookmasters